CURRICULAR
INJUSTICE

CURRICULAR INJUSTICE

HOW U.S. MEDICAL SCHOOLS REPRODUCE INEQUALITIES

LAUREN D. OLSEN

Columbia University Press   *New York*

Columbia University Press
Publishers Since 1893
New York   Chichester, West Sussex
cup.columbia.edu

Library of Congress Cataloging-in-Publication Data
Names: Olsen, Lauren D., author.
Title: Curricular injustice : how U.S. medical schools reproduce
inequalities / by Lauren D. Olsen, Assistant Professor, Department of
Sociology, College of Liberal Arts, Temple University.
Description: New York : Columbia University Press, 2024. |
Includes bibliographical references and index.
Identifiers: LCCN 2024002194 | ISBN 9780231207867 (hardback) |
ISBN 9780231207874 (trade paperback) | ISBN 9780231557153 (ebook)
Subjects: LCSH: Medical colleges—United States. | Discrimination in
medical care—United States. | Discrimination in medical
education—United States.
Classification: LCC R745 .O47 2024 | DDC 610.71/173—
dc23/eng/20240223
LC record available at https://lccn.loc.gov/2024002194

Printed and bound by CPI Group (UK) Ltd, Croydon, CR0 4YY

Cover design: Noah Arlow
Cover images: Shutterstock

CONTENTS

PREFACE

When I would tell people that I was studying how the U.S. medical profession was attempting to teach future physicians to be humane and equitable, most people expressed deep support for this curricular endeavor—that there was a *need*—even if they had mixed hope in the prospect. And invariably they had a story. They had a story about a time with a physician who was unpleasant, at best, or downright awful, at worst. I now share in this collective sentiment, having my own story or two, but when I started this project, I did not. As a child of two white physicians, I did not appreciate how rare my relatively pleasant experiences with physicians had been (and, when I am able to flex my social connections, still are). As I have a social background similar to that of many physicians, it was my witnessing of other people's experiences of inhumanities and inequities in the physician encounter that inspired this project.

In my first job after graduating from college as a religion major, I worked for a nonprofit in New York City oriented around providing social services for people with major mental illness. Here, I was struck by the cultural complexity of the human experience with mental illness and equally struck by how that complexity was excluded from consideration by physicians. Visit after visit, physicians edited out patients' experiences and prioritized pharmaceutical interventions over getting to know them. I wondered why physicians seemed uninterested in seeing their patients as people with vibrant inner lives. I hated how patients with Medicaid had far less options for care; how the intentions of patients of color were questioned; how patients who did not conform to cisnormative presentations of gender were met with less warmth; and how often physicians looked at me, the white cisgender woman with an Ivy League degree, to speak on behalf of the patient who was right in front of them.

I became curious about physician training. Fueling my interest further was what appeared to be a rather spirited discourse among physicians that extolled the virtues of "cultural competence." There was all this *talk* about needing to view patients holistically and getting to know patients from their own perspective, but there was very little *action* in the actual clinical encounters. I applied to graduate school because I wanted to know what physicians learned about culture, how understanding culture affected their professional identities and practices, and what happened along this bumpy road between talk and action. Thus, when I started this project as an early-career graduate student, I was both bothered by what I witnessed regarding patients' experiences with inhumane and inequitable healthcare and also optimistic that knowledge would rescue the medical profession from its health-care delivery problems.

My optimistic belief in knowledge-as-panacea was both abstract and specific. I believed in the abstract that if people—physicians, in this case—just knew better, they would act better. So many of the physicians I knew were wonderful people. If they simply knew about these patients' stories of rough clinical encounters, if they just understood about the unequal distribution of resources in U.S. society, then they would change their behavior and would work to change the profession. I believed specifically that lessons and perspectives from the humanities and social sciences, as encapsulated in some of the promise of cultural competence, would make physicians better equipped to deliver the kind of care their diverse patient population wanted and needed. My past optimism underscores a certain kind of dangerous ignorance that emanated from my privileged social background and was reinforced by my enculturation in institutions that upheld that same privileged position. Even in graduate school, it was easy to hold onto that kind of optimism—and in many ways I still do when I step into the classroom hoping to foster a learning environment that opens minds and, if going full tilt, transforms lives.

But in graduate school I also learned a more critical perspective of knowledge, with the ongoing and iterative thinking that happens through the close reading of texts, conversations with others, constructive feedback, data collection experiences, and writing. I also became more attuned to the processes by which structurally privileged actors and bodies of knowledge excluded, marginalized, and transformed structurally less privileged actors and ways of knowing. For example, I learned that the medical profession, just like other institutions within the United States, gained and maintained its professional power by directly (and indirectly) excluding nonwhite, nonmale, and nonelite students. I also learned that this same profession prided itself on producing "objective" or politically "neutral" knowledge—alongside an equally white, male, and elite academia— that pathologized nonwhite, nonmale, and nonelite patient populations and maligned scholarship and perspectives that challenged the status quo. I still have more to learn, I am sure, but in graduate school, I became captivated by what I call the *politics of knowledge application*, or the power struggles over whose voice counts in decisions over what knowledge is included (and excluded) in the values and practices of a professional workforce.

Within this context, I set out to study how the U.S. medical profession incorporated the humanities and social sciences into their curricular practices to make more humane and equitable physicians. And when I described this project to others during the data collection phase, I noticed that folks either lit up with that same optimistic belief in the power of knowledge to solve problems or they skeptically scoffed at the prospect of physicians caring about equity and empathy. By the time I was analyzing the data, I was fascinated by this space between naïve enthusiasm and hardened cynicism because so many of my respondents had impressions of their medical school's curricular practices that were much more complicated. I became more and more interested in what curricular practices accomplished, even if they failed to live up to their promises.

As the title of the book suggests, I ultimately became most concerned with *curricular injustice*, which in this case happens when medical educators—knowingly or not—enact curricular practices that maintain rather than ameliorate social inequalities. I conceptualize *curricular practices* as quite expansive, focusing on how the decisions that medical school leaders and educators make about *what* to include or exclude, as well as *who* to include or exclude, produce lessons that coalesce in contributing to upholding the medical profession as distinctly white and elite. To that latter end, I indicate in this book the race and gender of every participant when I introduce them. It might start to feel bulky or redundant because nearly every medical educator in a position of curricular power is white. But that's the point. My sample is representative of medical school leadership in the United States, and it is important to confront the privilege of who is in power at medical schools at every turn. At the least, that is a starting point.

LIST OF ABBREVIATIONS

AAMC: Association of American Medical Colleges
AHRQ: Agency on Healthcare Research and Quality
AMA: American Medical Association
CLAS: National Standards on Culturally and Linguistically Appropriate Services
FRAHME: Fundamental Role of the Arts and Humanities in Medical Education
GME: graduate medical education
HHC: Health Humanities Consortium
HHS-OMH: Department of Health and Human Services Office of Minority Health
IOM: Institute of Medicine
LCME: Liaison Committee on Medical Education
MCAT: Medical College Admission Test
MD: medical doctor
NASEM: National Academies of Sciences, Engineering, and Medicine
NEH: National Endowment for the Humanities
NICHD: National Institute of Child Health and Development
NIMH: National Institute of Mental Health
NSF: National Science Foundation
POM: practice of medicine

PRIME: Project to Rebalance and Integrate Medical Education
SHHV: Society for Health and Human Values
STEMM: science, technology, engineering, mathematics, and medicine
UME: undergraduate medical education
USMLE: United States Medical Licensing Exam

CURRICULAR INJUSTICE

INTRODUCTION

D r. Carley[1] was waiting for me perched on the steps leading into the building where she had her main campus office. A vibrant and warm white woman, she asked if I would be interested in walking a little farther to a place across the sprawling campus with better coffee. I had traveled a few hours that morning for the meeting, so I was happy to have some movement and caffeine myself. As we walked through the many buildings punctuated by beautiful gardens, Carley explained that, while she loved the coffee at this particular place, she also liked to build longer walks into her schedule because her days on campus were long and time for exercise often eluded her.

I had requested an interview with Carley because she is a physician and social scientist with a joint appointment in the medical school and liberal arts college at a large research university in the United States. I wanted to know how she and her colleagues incorporated the humanities and social sciences into their medical school's undergraduate medical education (UME) curriculum—that is, the first four years of allopathic medical school after which students receive the title of medical doctor (MD). We ended up speaking for hours. Despite possessing a résumé that would intimidate physicians and social scientists alike, Carley, an MD-PhD, exuded generosity and humility as we discussed her clinical work, research projects, teaching experiences, medical school's curricular practices, and impressions of the broader medical profession's approach to cultivating more humane and equitable physicians.

Carley had many curricular experiences to draw on, but at one point, she remarked that she had reservations about the way her well-intentioned colleagues prepared medical students to engage critically with social scientific knowledge. She recounted a story from her own teaching, one where she was trying to instruct medical students about the complexity of stereotyping—but felt like she failed. Carley started saying:

> It's funny—just today I got my evals from a lecture that I did at the medical school about this case that happened a long time ago in some of my earlier cancer work. There was a Latina woman. She had been diagnosed with cervical cancer and shuffled around all over the place. Doctors are always telling Latinas that they get cervical cancer because they've been sleeping around. So she asked this doctor right before surgery, "How come I got this?" And he said "Well, Anglos tend to get cancer of the breast more and Latinos tend to get cervical cancer." And she said "Why is that?" And the doctor tells her, "Because Anglos tend to smoke more and Latinos tend to start having sex at an earlier age and have more sexual partners."

At this point Carley paused and sipped her coffee, letting the setup of her example sink in. She then continued, noting that she "presented this case to the students *not* to say, like, 'look at this racist doctor,' but to say—'look at all of the training. He took his epidemiology on how you get cervical cancer or a sexually transmitted infection and then took the statistics that Latinos have higher rates of cervical cancer, and just smashed them together.'" Carley paused again and sighed. She went on to connect the dots for me, explaining how this one empirical example illustrated a broader pattern where physicians consuming social scientific knowledge without critical thinking yielded inaccuracies: "So it's one of those moments where you're taking all these things that you're learning and then come up with these ideas that are not right."

Much to Carley's chagrin, her overarching message about the hazards of decontextualized statistics was lost on the medical students in her class. She said to me:

> But the students—like students either love me or they hate me—the students that didn't like that conversation basically said that I just took this example of a racist doctor. "We all know that he's racist," and just went off with that. That's not what happened, but it's interesting that that's their perception of what happened. Because they're not seeing the value of the conversation on how easily that *could* happen. They don't need to be a racist; it's going to happen to all of them. They're all getting taught the same things and one day they're going to say something stupid like that.
>
> Does that mean they're racist? Well, I think we're all a little racist. But the goal wasn't to say look at all these racists. The goal was to help them think about how easily these things—stereotyping, misdiagnosis, overlooking a diagnosis—happen. So I think for those students that example was a failure. It made me think about how I can do this differently so that I get at those students that don't get it right away.

In Carley's one opportunity within her medical school's limited curricular time devoted to teaching about social inequalities, her attempt to teach students about critical approaches to consuming and applying social scientific knowledge fell flat.

She *was* trying, though. And her medical school was, too. Despite trying, Carley felt like she failed. Her account was but one among many I heard throughout the course of my research about the varieties of curricular failures that frustrated medical educators—clinicians, humanists, and social scientists alike—as they attempted to train future physicians to engage in humane and equitable care. These failures happened despite good intentions. They happened despite there being *at least some* opportunities for integrating social scientific and humanistic content into curricular practices. Their delivery was stymied by a host of limitations, some of which were featured in Carley's example: medical students were fixated on the racist individual and unable to see how racism was embedded into knowledge systems; most clinical faculty members routinely taught decontextualized information about social groups;[2] UME leaders designing the curriculum allotted only one session in the entire four years of training for a nonbiomedical or nonclinical subject; students were not equipped to value these conversations; and individual educators were often the ones responsible for improving the delivery of this content.

In this book, I describe how the medical profession, in its attempt to integrate the humanities and social sciences to develop humane and equitable future physicians, often failed to do so, resulting in curricular injustice. Clinical faculty members, in their capacity as curricular designers and implementers, were at the heart of these failures. Their limited understandings of the critical and reflective contributions of these fields patterned their delivery of the material. Failure happened at each step in the *process of knowledge application*, which in this particular case was their process of transforming the potential of the humanities and social sciences into actual curricular practices in medical school classrooms.

From their decisions about placement within the overall curriculum to choices about what substantive content to include and exclude from these fields of knowledge, clinical faculty members' good intentions were rarely realized. Instead, medical students received lessons about how the social sciences and humanities could be relevant for clinical practice—but in ways that continued to implicate the medical profession in the creation and maintenance of social inequalities, as Carley's opening example illustrates. Thus, this book matters for our understanding of how medical educators—and perhaps educators and professionals more broadly—make decisions that continue to uphold the white, elite status quo of their profession while dismissing, marginalizing, or problematizing the people and ideas that deviate from it. And the stakes are high, with humane and equitable care on the line. While this is mostly a book about these good intentions, about these limited understandings, and ultimately about the dangers that flowed from this perilous pairing, I also show that it does not need to be this way. Indeed, there is hope for the future of UME emanating from the few schools where educators got it right.

CURRICULAR PROMISES AND PROBLEMS

Curricular reform teems of promise. Change the curriculum, change the training, change the profession, change the world. The curricular-reform-to-global-change pipeline is not, of course, so straightforward. The *potential* that reform holds, however, remains an important tenet of white liberalism. White liberalism is one of the historically and contemporarily dominant political approaches in the United States that promotes the application of expert knowledge to solve social problems through incremental reform.[3] Curricular reform involving the humanities and social sciences also holds a specific progressive potential wrapped up in how these bodies of knowledge are associated with promises of fostering equity and enriching humanity.[4]

National calls for integrating the humanities and social sciences into biomedical fields blossomed at the close of the twentieth century in the United States, with federal agencies like the National Science Foundation (NSF), National Academies of Sciences, Engineering, and Medicine (NASEM), and the National Endowment of the Humanities (NEH) all publishing reports and recommendations about the need for the humanities and social sciences to be integrated into science, technology, engineering, mathematics, and medicine (STEMM) fields.[5] The nationwide efforts also had some teeth. These federal agencies—in addition to private and professional organizations—underwrote training programs and ushered in curricular developments in STEMM education. With these kinds of investments, leaders of professional education viewed the integration of the social sciences and humanities into STEMM and clinical training as important for building professional knowledge, skills, and attitudes. From these curricular initiatives in medical education, a profile emerged of physicians: they should know their patients' social context and hone their critical, interpretive, and observational knowledge and skills for the clinic. They should be socially accountable.[6]

In addition to national, profession-wide calls for curricular reform, reform initiatives within the U.S. medical profession also occurred at the individual school level, shown in the case discussed by Dr. Carley. With school-initiated curricular reforms, medical educators at individual schools innovated a set of curricular practices that they documented, evaluated, and presented at national conferences, like the Association of American Medical Colleges (AAMC) annual meeting, and wrote about in professional journals, like *Academic Medicine*. Regardless of the origin—top-down initiatives from profession-wide bodies such as the AAMC and the Liaison Committee on Medical Education (LCME) or bottom-up initiatives at particular schools—individual schools enacted them. Each school, therefore, was an organization that contributed to the reproduction of the profession by either developing curricular practices of their own or adopting, interpreting, and implementing the professional standards and programming.

With regard to top-down initiatives, the AAMC and LCME explicitly encouraged the inclusion of the humanities and social sciences into the UME.[7] With the social sciences, the LCME standards *mandated* that medical educators instruct students about the manifestations and underpinnings of social inequalities in the first four years of medical school; otherwise, the medical school could risk losing its accreditation. The required curricular content from the LCME standards contained material from several social science fields, especially those related to individual and population health, implicit bias, and the health-care delivery process, but there were no requirements in place demanding faculty members be hired or trained in specific social science disciplines.[8]

With the exception of bioethics, the humanities were not required for accreditation; however, the AAMC made the humanities a priority, funding a new initiative, the Fundamental Role of Arts and Humanities in Medical Education (FRAHME).[9] This initiative ran on the heels of the Project to Rebalance and Integrate Medical Education (PRIME) at the AAMC, wherein educators hoped to utilize the humanities to promote empathy, virtue, genuineness, and self-awareness.[10] While not mandated like the social sciences, there has been a profession-wide adoption of some sort of humanities content into curricular practices. For example, in 2016, there were fifty-seven health humanities programs at U.S. medical schools, up from just fourteen in 2000.[11] Similarly, in 2016, 94 percent of medical schools participating in a survey (N = 134, which is just three schools shy of the accredited MD-granting schools in that year) had either required or elective humanities courses, with elective courses nearly doubling in the span of just four years.[12]

And yet, as historical precedent and sociological theory have shown again and again—and Carley's account demonstrates—the enactment of curricular reform does not always go as planned.[13] In my study, clinical faculty members overwhelmingly agreed with the importance of teaching medical students the lessons from the humanities and social sciences. When I interviewed medical educators about what they taught, I started with broad questions about when and where it was taught. Medical educators would pull out curricular maps, and even though they often struggled to explain curricular practices in detail, they were enthusiastic about the need for learning this material. Students told a far less enthusiastic story.

In general, medical students reported that they received limited content from social sciences and that it was up to them to engage with the humanities. Students felt that their clinical faculty members were ill-equipped to facilitate instruction in these fields, with students carping about how clinical faculty often had patients or students talk about their lived experience as the way to learn the social science material, or they had students run book clubs so that they might have a humanities elective. From the students' perspective, social science curricula were rendered meaningless, were reduced in complexity, and were often relegated solely to the realm of experience despite being a LCME-mandated curricular requirement. Based on students' remarks, the humanities curricula were treated as a space for students to cope with the discontents of medical school or to shore up their white elite pedigree. The medical educators' ameliorative curricular dreams did not translate into the curricular practices that they hoped them to be—and sometimes the failure further entrenched the kinds of equity and empathy problems that the profession was trying to address in the first place.

PRIOR EXPLANATIONS OF CURRICULAR REFORM FAILURE

How do these curricular dreams fail? When I began my research, I found three potential explanations from different subfields within sociology. The first explanation comes from medical sociology, with scholars questioning the intentions of the medical profession's desire to enact meaningful change. The second explanation comes from organizational sociology, whereby sociologists illuminated the difficulties that accompanied reform efforts within organizations, like medical schools. The third explanation comes from science and technology scholars who studied the power imbalances between biomedical scientists, on the one hand, and humanists and social scientists, on the other. Each of these explanations helps tell part of the story—but not the whole story because each one lacks some key components to the curricular reform failure puzzle.

The first explanation was the closest to the empirical case and came from medical sociologists bemoaning the failure of previous curricular reforms within medical education. Samuel Bloom was a medical sociologist who dedicated much of his career to the inclusion of the social sciences in U.S. medical schools. Early in his career, in the late 1950s and into the 1960s, he was moderately successful in his curricular efforts; by the 1970s, however, he felt that social science—and social scientists—were marginalized within medical education.[14] One of his central explanations was that the reimbursement structure of the medical school rendered any inclusions of social science as merely token because clinical faculty members were not incentivized to focus on teaching when most of their income came from their research or clinical work. These schools often engaged in what he described as "reform without change," pointing to the public relations work that the invocation of "reform" achieved at the expense of any meaningful change.[15]

Other medical sociologists were also wary and critical of what they felt were public relations campaigns dressed up as caring about including the social sciences. Both Howard Waitzkin and Donald Light have discussed the impossibility for the social sciences to be applied critically without an entire overhaul of the material commitments of U.S. medical schools and health care writ large. Their skepticism was not overblown, as Waitzkin had first-hand experience with the marginalization of his field (and position) after being pushed out of a medical school for daring to teach critical social sciences in the context of medical education.[16] Light has argued further that any inclusion of social science into medical education would compromise the critical capacity of social scientists because they would cease to retain their outside position.[17] Taken together, these explanations of curricular reform failure questioned the integrity of the medical profession's intentions regarding incorporating new curricular practices.

A second set of scholars poised to explain why these curricular reforms failed come from organizational sociology. These scholars took up the question of reform failure across organizations, documenting the extent and varieties of how standards were decoupled—that is, disconnected from, not followed, or only partially applied—from the day-to-day practices in organizations (e.g., a firm or a school).[18] These scholars offer many insights that explain failure, especially that of "symbolic compliance." With symbolic compliance, Lauren Edelman demonstrated that the more opaque a standard—and thus the less specific the instructions on how to enact the standard and the less specific the consequences should that standard not be implemented—the more likely the organizational actors responsible for implementing the standard would comply only symbolically.[19] As opposed to the medical sociologists' focus on the structure of medical schools, many of these organizational sociologists explained the discrepancies between standard and practice by examining the cultural norms on the ground inhibiting the reform efforts.[20] Scholars have also implicated the informal processes in place that normalize deviance within the established operational protocols, in turn yielding a functional incoherence to the organization.[21] For example, as sociologist Katherine Kellogg has shown, if there is an informal culture at a hospital that glorifies or normalizes overwork, then implementing a patient safety reform curtailing work hours could be difficult to achieve.[22]

The third potential explanation for curricular reform failure stems from an interdisciplinary body of work on the distribution of power between biomedical disciplines, on the one hand, and humanities and social sciences, on the other. These scholars described the power imbalances built into the structures of academic and healthcare institutions that put more resources in the hands of biomedical and clinical faculty. They also pointed to the cultures of positivism and neoliberalism that permeated these institutions, cultures that rewarded the pursuit of "objective," "useful," and "monetizable" knowledge. They contended that the structure and culture of academic and healthcare institutions created the conditions under which the social sciences and humanities were perpetually undervalued.[23] Drawing on ethnographic research of collaborations between biomedical, humanist, and social scientist actors engaged in scientific research projects, these scholars described biomedical actors as holding disdain, disregard, or dislike for the humanities and social sciences. In other words, they depicted biomedical scientists holding "epistemic hostility" toward their nonbiomedical peers, which sometimes took the form of exclusion, sometimes as appropriation, or sometimes as care work.[24] These researchers also identified different cultural markers of interdisciplinary collaboration success: humanists and social scientists believed interdisciplinary integration was successful when students adopted a critical awareness, whereas biomedical scientists believed integration was successful if their team collaborated well.[25]

Each of these bodies of work informs the present story. I am wary of the dubious intentions of a profession's discursive calls for curricular reform. I am curious about the organizational barriers that complicate the everyday implementation of profession-wide programming. I am attuned to the epistemic hostility that social scientists and humanists might meet in their encounters with colleagues from biomedicine. But a few key observations from my study made these lines of explanation incomplete.

First, these white scholars treated professions and organizations— and the actors within them—as socially neutral. While social inequalities were an outcome of some of these studies, race, gender, class, and sexuality did not figure into their analyses, and a growing number of scholars have illuminated how these assumptions of professional and social homogeneity within the medical profession are major oversights.[26] To grasp the failures of these curricular reform efforts fully, a greater understanding is needed about the organizational processes that have kept white clinical faculty members in positions of power— and the epistemic limitations of the white, elite, Western biomedical knowledge that they wield. Therefore, in this book, I contextualize the medical profession's historical and contemporary approach to curricular practices with critical race, postcolonial, and feminist work.[27]

Second, the clinical faculty members in my study seemed to have a genuine wish to include the humanities and social sciences—as

Carley demonstrated in the opening example, they were *trying*. With the prior explanations, scholars tended to overlook the *applied* biomedical actors' perspectives and actions, specifically those of the clinical faculty members. In my study, clinical faculty members saw value in the social sciences and humanities, witnessing and experiencing a need for the incorporation of these fields; in fact, some claimed that previous epistemic hostility to humanistic and social scientific knowledge might be abating. Thus, while there may have been some clinical faculty members who were hostile, most in my study perceived themselves to be quite welcoming. In my explanation of curricular reform failure throughout this book, I show how most clinical faculty members fundamentally misunderstood these fields and how they could relate to health and health care.

My final key observation was oriented around the effects of curricular reform failure. I agree with previous scholars that the medical profession's calls for meaningful curricular change were not borne out in the enacted practices at each medical school. But contrary to prior work that focused on these decoupled practices as merely symbolic, I found that curricular practices, even if they were failures, *did* achieve learning outcomes—just not the ones that were imagined in the first place. In addition to focusing on the consequences of seemingly innocuous curricular failures, I also draw attention to how medical leaders created the conditions to encourage organizational decoupling. The gap between the standard and the enacted practice was posited as a professional oversight problem. I argue, however, that to truly appreciate the contours of curricular reform failure, a school's organizational flexibility must be understood as a *formal* source of professional power rather than an *informal* accident. The medical profession built the conditions for decoupling into the process of knowledge application by giving individual schools the latitude to interpret these standards.

As I will show throughout the book, I push the scholarly conversations further by focusing on the function that curricular practices play in reifying power and inequalities within professions and organizations. It was not just a publicity stunt because the curriculum was productive and physicians were invested; it was not just exclusion because the curriculum captured many different relationships between the humanities, social sciences, and biomedicine; and it was not just inadvertent decoupling because organizational flexibility was pivotal to professional power.

WHERE GOOD INTENTIONS MEET LIMITED UNDERSTANDINGS

My observations raised a new puzzle: why do curricular reforms continue to fail even with the buy-in and enthusiasm of clinical faculty members? How can we explain the disconnect between discourse (e.g., articulated intentions and values) and implementation (e.g., practices and understandings) in the medical profession's quest to improve patient care by including the humanities and social sciences in its curricular practices? I advance an answer that centers on the clinical faculty's *limited understandings* of the humanities and social sciences. As the central designers and executors of curricular practices, clinical faculty members were integral to interpreting the AAMC programming guidelines and LCME standards, evaluating humanities and social sciences knowledge for their relevance, and enacting these understandings in decisions about curricular practices. This included what was taught; when and how it was taught; who taught it; and, of course, what and who were excluded from these curricular practices. Even if they approached curricular reform with enthusiasm, they produced curricular practices that failed to live up to their promise.

A few fundamental points about the organizational, moral, and epistemic components of the medical profession—and their reproductive units, medical schools—influenced how clinical faculty members came to interpret, evaluate, and enact the humanities and social sciences within their UME curricular practices. These components about the medical profession are symbolic and pragmatic expressions of power, revealing how medical schools continue to produce a particular view of the world and the physician's place within it. And while I tease apart the organizational, moral, and epistemic components for the sake of clarity, they are nevertheless overlapping and mutually inform one another. Their combination limits the clinical faculty members' understanding of the critical and interpretive capacities of the humanities and social sciences.

First, the organizational structure of medical schools is fragmented, confusing, and in a perpetual state of "crisis." The incoherence and flexibility had a few instantiations: vague professional standards (e.g., LCME standards), splintered surroundings (e.g., scattered buildings), segmented positions (e.g., percentage time on clinic, teaching, administration), hierarchical relationships (e.g., attending, resident, medical student), overwhelming schedules (e.g., high-patient load, performance standards, resource scarcity), and individual choice for medical students (e.g., pathways, concentrations). Many educators voiced a resigned belief in this disorganization, which is important as it obscured the fact that leaders were, indeed, making decisions that affected curricular reform. Most medical school leaders have a similar overarching approach to governing medical education, prioritizing research and clinical activities over teaching, all while extracting as much labor from their faculty as possible. Leaders engage in haphazard hiring processes and cobble together part-time, temporary medical education positions, decisions that by and large place white clinical faculty members in positions of curricular power and promote siloed problem-solving.[28]

Following organizational scholars, I found it helpful to conceptualize medical schools as "organized anarchies" because there is a functionality to the incoherence, a logic to the flexibility.[29] While a source for curricular reform failure, a school's *organizational flexibility* is also a source of power; organizational flexibility is a medical school leadership's mechanism for absorbing critique and discouraging systematic curricular change. While medical schools are organized in ways that put clinical faculty members in positions of power, these faculty members are not set up for curricular reform success. There are simply not enough hours in a day, week, month, year for clinical faculty members to accomplish everything they need to accomplish. They juggle multiple responsibilities at once, from in-class teaching to clinical rounding, to seeing patients, to research, to writing grants, to seemingly endless administrative work. Under these organizational conditions, clinical faculty members do not have much time to dedicate to curricular design and instruction. Not only do they have little time to immerse themselves in, engage with, and learn new subject matter, but there is also less time for critical appraisal.

Second, the moral framing of the medical profession further obscures reflexivity and critique. Central to the medical profession's self-concept, or professional identity, is that physicians are *good*. They are doctors, for goodness' sake! They are "the best of the best," to quote one of my respondents.[30] They save lives, improve health— they even have a ceremony that celebrates and symbolizes their sanctity and purity, where they don their white coats and recite the Hippocratic Oath.[31] Their efficacy and advancements certainly cannot be understated, but this moral framing that lionizes the profession as altruistic, apolitical, and amazing creates a certain attitude that I call *Hippocratic hubris*.

Placed on a pedestal, physicians are instilled with confidence that they are in the best profession and deserve all the entitlement that comes with it. As other scholars have shown, clinical faculty members are treated like the paramount experts and health-care providers— they often come across like they think they know everything and their knowledge and work are more important than that of others.[32] Sociologists have aided in this construction, too, as sociologist LaTonya Trotter has insightfully argued—Talcott Parsons and Robert Merton glorified the medical profession with their agenda-setting (at the time) accounts, and sociologists continue to center the medical profession and marginalize other health-care professions.[33] I am guilty of centering physicians, as well. As with other professions oriented around an altruistic mission, this moral framing shrouds physicians in "an aura of benevolent power," making it difficult for members of the profession to grapple with their racist, classist, paternalistic, and cis- and heteronormative views.[34] This Hippocratic hubris obscures the scope of the profession's complicity with and contributions to inequality while arming its members with the confidence that they are on the right side of history.[35] To be fair, academic professions are also implicated in similar moral framing processes that cloud their self-concept and approach to equity.

Third, the epistemic orientation of the medical profession elevates white clinical faculty members as the experts par excellence and constrains their understanding of the humanities and social sciences. The medical profession's belief in the "superiority of clinical experience"[36] and the white Western positivist tradition locates expertise squarely within the domain of the physician. Those who adhere to this positivist tradition believe that there is a "Cartesian knower" or "modest witness" who objectively observes a phenomenon and can accurately report "just the facts" based on what they see.[37] As scholars like Julian Go have drawn attention to and critiqued, this objective observer and consummate expert professional is most certainly code for white.[38] And while historically constructed, it remains socially real today that scientific excellence is *still* understood as the domain of white men and that anecdotal experience comes from people of color and women.[39]

In addition to the importance of understanding *who* knows, it is also crucial to spell out *what is being known*. In the latter half of the twentieth century, the facts that clinical faculty members knew and learned were overwhelmingly biomedical in nature as part of the reign of the "bio-bio-bio" approach,[40] or the approach that biomedical knowledge could explain and solve all health problems. As a result, the bulk of the early twenty-first century clinical faculty leadership in

U.S. medical schools have minimal, if any, training in the social sciences and humanities. They came of age when "the social" had been constructed as external to the medical profession. If anything, "the social" was incorporated as the "art" of medicine in direct contrast to the "science" of medicine.[41] Thus, even as the dominance of bio-bio-bio models abated, the clinical faculty members charged with incorporating social sciences and humanities knowledge into the newer "bio-psy-soc" models for interacting and evaluating patients did not have training in how to go about this task.[42] This generational lag has yielded a limited, superficial, or inaccurate engagement with these bodies of knowledge.

While clinical faculty members have gaps in their expertise about structural inequalities and critical appraisals of their field, what they *do* have is vast clinical experience. This prism of clinical experience influences how they understand the value of the humanities and social sciences. With the humanities, the clinical faculty members' experiences with the difficulties and discontents within clinical practice—what I call empathy problems—primed them to appreciate the humanities for their therapeutic and celebratory capacities. They centered themselves and their experiences—as opposed to other health-care workers and patients—in how they envisioned the humanities' relevance for physicians, in turn leaving out the critical and reflective contributions of these fields.

Against this backdrop of accumulated clinical experience, with the social sciences, clinical faculty members struggled to see beyond the individual as the unit of analysis; they struggled to see the scale of structural inequalities.[43] The individual is the epistemic object of clinical attention, with physicians seeing one patient at a time;[44] these experiences made clinical faculty see the importance of "the social," but they could not see beyond the frame of the singular patient and their "anecdotes." The primacy of clinical experience for clinical faculty in positions of curricular power folded together moral, expert, paternalistic, and white authority, coalescing into what I call *clinical witnessing.* Clinical witnessing entails faculty appreciating the existence of health and health-care inequalities as "clinically relevant" problems—what I call equity problems—through witnessing patients' individual accounts of them.

Amid the organizational flexibility, Hippocratic hubris, and clinical witnessing, the clinical faculty members had an ever-increasing awareness of empathy and equity problems but not a critical or reflective understanding of them. Despite their good intentions, medical educators operated as if they were on a hamster wheel of white liberal curricular reform. White liberal curricular reform is premised on the notion that "society is meliorative—gradually moving toward perfection—through incremental reforms or social action," which Louise Seamster and Victor Ray refer to as the "progress paradigm."[45] Importantly, the clinical faculty members' incremental steps—cherry-picking bits and pieces of the social sciences and humanities fields in service of clinical relevance—are not just serving the medical profession. These incremental steps that do not address the root problems are also indicative of the profession's "possessive investment in whiteness," whether the clinical faculty members are aware of it or not.[46] Their ignorance is active and dynamic.[47]

THE DANGEROUS IMPLICATIONS OF LIMITED UNDERSTANDINGS

By constraining the design and instruction, clinical faculty's limited understandings manifested in curricular design and implementation choices that affected how students valued humanistic and social scientific information. When the clinical faculty members decided to include the humanities as electives, they signaled to students that these fields were external to what physicians *really* needed to know. When clinical faculty members celebrated white "canonical" texts and elite art forms, they presented and platformed a specific social identity. When they encouraged students to engage with the humanities for therapeutic purposes, they taught them how to cope with—rather than challenge—the professional status quo.

The way that clinical faculty members approached the instruction of social sciences also had impacts on what students appreciated. For instance, many clinical faculty members decided to teach the social sciences in a one-week intersession before a break when students were about to leave for the holidays. Many clinical faculty members also conscripted students of color to talk about their experiences in small-group discussions as the only time students learned about race. When they did include content in lectures, clinical faculty members drew on social scientific knowledge that was delimited to decontextualized statistics or individual stories. These choices combined to obscure critical and structural knowledge about the origins, legacies, and reach of social inequalities.

In structuring the courses and delivering the problematic content in the classroom, clinical faculty reached for lessons that assumed, reinforced, and glorified a conflation of the professional clinician with the white elite. This approach reified who were objects and who were subjects. Patients, nonwhite people, poor people, "socially complex" people, and queer people were objects. Clinicians, white people, elite people, and straight people were subjects. Objects were to be known; subjects mattered. While it may seem simple and obvious in terms of explicit learning outcomes, it was a curricular injustice that medical students did not think that they needed to care about racism or know the appropriate gender pronouns to use for patients. It was a curricular injustice that students thought that the humanities were just useful for their own catharsis or to showcase a set of talents from the white upper class rather than a robust set of critical and reflective knowledge that could improve how physicians approached patient care.

More implicit lessons were also conveyed through these curricular practices; more subtle socialization occurred. In this sense, it was also a curricular injustice that students were taught to stay quiet and take care of their own mental health, that their peers were all like effortless concert pianists, that they were suckers if they really cared about the underserved, that social science was just anecdotal, that it was up to them to learn about structural inequalities. It was also a curricular injustice that students of color were differentially treated in their coursework and clerkships—in terms of both their temporal and emotional taxation—relative to their white peers. As I will show in this book, the clinical faculty members' limited understandings produced docile workers via reinforcing the status quo, promoted the devolution of responsibility to individuals, taxed identities and reified stereotypes, maintained social inequalities by focusing on anecdotes rather than structural problems, and lacked a reflexivity regarding the power relations in the medical profession.[48]

By illuminating the curricular practices informing how students learned to approach patient care, I contribute to our broader understanding of how physicians engage in inequitable and inhumane care in the first place. In other words, other scholars' empirical research suggests that the curricular decisions outlined in this book could have serious ramifications for socially marginalized patients down the line. For example, in one recent study, white male physicians were more likely to be a risk to patient safety than physicians of color and some white female physicians.[49] In another set of studies, scholars demonstrated that when physicians are confused about race or gender, they are more likely to engage in biased care.[50] In yet another study, scholars showed that physicians drew on problematic approaches to social science (e.g., cultural stereotypes, individual-level implicit bias) to feel absolved from wrongdoing.[51]

In addition to patient outcomes, with medical education programs like the Healer's Art and E.M.P.A.T.H.Y., entrepreneurially inclined physicians are transforming the humanities and social sciences to make a profit.[52] This entrepreneurial approach is akin to "health equity tourism," which Elle Lett's team defines as "the practice of investigators—without prior experience or commitment to health equity research—parachuting into the field in response to timely and often temporary increases in public interest and resources."[53] Therefore, with the expansion of these nonbiomedical curricular practices into medical education, there could also be an attendant medicalization and commodification of the humanities and social sciences, which may be serving the interests of this entrepreneurial class more than the patient population. As Lett and colleagues argue, this entrepreneurial spirit has implications for both knowledge production and application—to use their language, not only does the influx of these "tourists" hungry for research funding "pollute" the health equity field with inaccurate and potentially damaging work, but it also "dilutes" the impact of the important work already being done by researchers committed to health justice.[54]

Building off that latter point, the observations contained in this book are thus also instructive for our broader understandings of the politics of knowledge application and curricular reform in U.S. professions, organizations, and institutions. The curriculum—as an outcome of a set of decisions about what to include and what to exclude, where to put it, how to teach it, who should do the teaching, and how to test it—is an outcome of a set of power relations reflecting the values and attitudes of the leaders of a profession.[55] While the empirical case contained in this book focuses on the medical profession, these kinds of choices are being made elsewhere. Just like with leaders of the medical profession, university leaders are making choices with their organizational processes around curricular reform—about who is at the table and what is being discussed at that table. University leaders are making choices about how they design and execute diversity, equity, and inclusion practices but also about how they decide what the general education requirements for *all* their undergraduates should be.[56] These kinds of choices are also being made by other professional training programs, like police, law, or business.[57] Curricular practices, therefore, capture the general social process by which professions, organizations, and institutions shape orientations toward inequality itself.

THE HUMANITIES AND SOCIAL SCIENCES IN UNDERGRADUATE MEDICAL EDUCATION

To study how leaders of U.S. medical schools attempted to incorporate the humanities and social sciences into their curricular practices to cultivate humane and equitable future physicians, I collected data from 2015 through 2017. I started at the profession-wide level, gathering reports and standards put out by professional organizations, such as the AAMC and LCME. To situate the project, I tracked how medical educators understood the role of the humanities and social sciences in training the physician over the course of the twentieth century as captured in their central journal, what is now known as *Academic Medicine*, and with historians' accounts. I then examined twenty-first-century profession-wide discussions both in print and at several national pedagogical meetings, such as the AAMC annual meeting on medical education. I found the question-and-answer period following presentations to be the most illuminating about the tensions and opportunities present when educators attempt to integrate the social sciences and humanities into their UME curricular practices.

As I moved from the profession-wide discourse about UME curricular practices to the enactment of them at the level of an individual school, I gathered a set of curricular materials (e.g., curricular maps, course descriptions) from all 137 accredited MD-granting medical schools within the United States at the time. While some medical schools provided reams of curricular information, replete with syllabi, lesson plans, assessments, and evaluations, there were two main categories of data that were pertinent and available at each medical school. The first were the descriptions of each course in years 1, 2, 3, and 4. These course descriptions contained the title of the course and what was taught in it. The second category of information was the curricular map. These schematic representations indicated how much time was dedicated to a particular topic and when it was taught.

Taken together, these data captured curricular requirements, electives, and extracurricular programming.

To better understand how medical educators made decisions about UME curricular practices—both in terms of what to teach when and in terms of their approaches to in-classroom instruction—I interviewed medical educators from different professional and disciplinary backgrounds. I also interviewed medical students to appreciate how they received their schools' curricular practices. In total, I interviewed thirty medical students and sixty medical educators (thirty with a clinical background, thirty with (at least) a humanities or social sciences background) from thirty-seven different medical schools. The central objective for interviewing people from these groups was to leverage comparisons across fields (e.g., clinical, humanities, social sciences) and across status (e.g., faculty member, student). The interviews allowed the "official" arbiters of medical education reform and design to describe how they developed and evaluated curricular practices, why they wanted (or did not want) to include the humanities and social sciences in their curricular practices, and what the humanities and social sciences meant to them. The interviews with educators allowed them to explain some of the opportunities and challenges that had an impact on their curricular efforts, describing the curriculum they would ideally have compared to what they were able to implement, and the discrepancies that arose between the two. In contrast, the interviews with the medical students provided a window into what the "official" consumers of curricular practices learned about the humanities and social sciences—both how it was taught and how it was situated relative to the rest of their training.[58]

My analytical approach was an iterative process of triangulating between data sources. With the historical, curricular, and observational data, I situated the successes, failures, constructions of the relevance of humanistic and social scientific knowledge for medicine, and negotiations of interdisciplinary work within the broader social, cultural, interprofessional, and organizational environment. With the interviews, I identified contemporary conceptualizations of the value of the humanities and social sciences for clinical practice, the challenges and opportunities that educators from different fields faced in attempting to collaborate in incorporating this knowledge into medical education, and the overall impressions of the success and failure of their attempts. I often fought—mostly myself—to keep the humanities in this analysis because, despite the elective status of the humanities, its contribution to a holistic set of understandings was too important for the overall curricular injustice story. For more information on my data and methodology, please refer to the methodological appendix.

PLAN OF THE BOOK

Wrapped up in the opening account with Dr. Carley were a host of considerations that I take up in this book. For one, the account showed the effort and intentions on behalf of a medical educator trying to cultivate a critical consciousness in students and the carved-out curricular space to do so. Despite the opportunities, Carley's account also illustrated the perils of positivistic, decontextualized approaches to social science and the epistemic barriers that critical knowledge was up against in medical education. Carley's experience also presented organizational barriers, highlighting how the variable and fragmented organizational structure of UME rendered so much of this instruction up to the practices of individual educators, as she pondered, "How can *I* do this differently?" This example also exhibited the potential for curricular futility because if this were the only time that students were given an opportunity to learn about this material then the pedagogical outcome was much less likely to be effective.

To unfurl the moving parts, I have organized the chapters in a processual arrangement, showing the process of knowledge application. Chapter 1 is a starting point in which I highlight the history of how the social sciences and humanities were incorporated into U.S. medical education in the twentieth century. In the first half of the twentieth century, leaders of the medical profession largely incorporated the humanities in what I call an *inclusion-as-admissions* approach by admitting students who had backgrounds in the humanities as a proxy for their class and racial background. They also incorporated the humanities and then the social sciences in an *inclusion-as-integration* approach, where educators included knowledge from these fields into the curricular practices. In chapter 1, I make the case for why curricular practices are productive and ideological by focusing on what leaders of the profession thought physicians needed to know and who physicians needed to be.

In chapter 2, I bring the discussion into the twenty-first century and center the contemporary professional conversations about curricular reform in medicine. Here, leaders in medical education dreamed about wielding the social sciences and humanities disciplines to solve the *equity problems* and *empathy problems* that the U.S. medical profession faced, from social inequalities to burnout. These dreams were well intentioned, but they were also quite vague. Therefore, in chapter 3, I detail how the profession-wide curricular dreams were interpreted by the clinical faculty members who oversaw the design of curricular practices at their individual medical schools. As I move from the profession level to the organization level, I show how organizational and epistemic barriers coalesced to marginalize the social sciences and humanities in the curricular practices of most medical schools.

In chapter 4, I draw attention to the particular problems that occurred with instruction, which emanated from the clinical faculty members' limited expertise with the social sciences and humanities. These were not neutral problems but rather curricular injustices—the clinical faculty engaged in curricular practices that were inaccurate, placating, and unequal. For example, faculty had students of color teach their peers about race by sharing their lived experience, in what I call the *conscripted curriculum*; they had students engage in a book club as a means to address the burnout that their current and future selves (would) face. As a result, these clinical faculty members often established a contrast between the "facts" learned from physicians and the "experience" learned from the lives of students and patients, producing what I call the *anecdotalization effect.* In chapter 5, I turn my attention to how this compounded failure affected the medical students, and the ideological socialization that occurred based on what they learned and what was left out.

In the conclusion, I illustrate the exceptions to this process—the few schools that did not engage in these varieties of curricular failure and instead cultivated a critical consciousness in their students. There is hope yet! This hope inheres in a medical school's *intellectual infrastructure*, or scholars who have expertise in the humanities and social sciences and have power over the design and instruction of curricular practices. I conclude with a discussion of what we can learn from these successes and failures and advance several policy recommendations. Curricular change that has a lasting impact on reducing inequalities cannot be achieved without physicians having a solid grasp of the historical underpinnings and structural manifestations of social inequalities, and grappling with their profession's role in perpetuating and participating in many of these racist, classist, paternalistic, and cis- and heteronormative systems.

1

CURRICULAR PRACTICES
AND PROFESSIONAL POWER

Carlyle Jacobsen performed the first prefrontal lobotomy on a chimpanzee in 1935. As he rose in prominence, he grew and innovated medical education for the State University of New York (SUNY). In addition to spearheading the incorporation of radiation and x-ray technologies into educational programming for SUNY, he was also integral to national conversations about medical school admissions and curricular practices. In 1949, the same year that Egaz Moniz won a Nobel Prize for the lobotomy on humans, in a discussion at the meeting of the Association of American Medical Colleges (AAMC), Jacobsen focused the participants' attention on two interrelated questions: what constitutes a good medical student, and how can those good students be identified in the admissions process?

The discussion was fruitful, if not bordering on redundant. As Jacobsen remarked, "[I]n the course of commenting on the academic, it was said again and again, 'well, we want the well-rounded man.'" He continued, "there were varying ways of describing this individual, but obviously it was not a dullard who was wanted, but somebody who was interested in affairs of life, as well as the pure intellectual activity."[1] "Well-rounded" physicians have been the order of the day in professional medicine from Jacobsen's time to the present.[2] While some progress has been made in terms of social representation in the medical profession, Jacobsen's wishes still ring true all these decades later: the U.S. medical profession remains dominated by well-rounded white men, where well-roundedness is a proxy for class—and racial—background.[3]

Evidence from admissions data suggests that medical schools select students from the white and elite segments of society, although equity-oriented improvement has been made with regard to gender.[4] In 1959 and 1960, women received 6 percent of medical degrees in the United Stares. By 1989 and 1990, their share of degrees increased to 34 percent, and by 2018, they held around 50 percent of all medical degrees. While there is parity in entering the profession, this parity begins to diminish as women advance in their careers. With every step along the career ladder (e.g., attendings, chairs, deans), men become overrepresented.[5] There is also very limited national data on gender identity and sexuality within the U.S. physician workforce, but with the smaller studies that have been conducted, scholars note that the profession is overwhelmingly cis- and hetero-normative in composition and culture.[6]

With regard to race, in 1964, 97 percent of the medical profession was white, and by 2018, 52 percent of the profession was white, but medical students who identify as Black or Latinx remain underrepresented, each comprising roughly 6 percent of incoming medical students. The leadership structure paints a similar, albeit worse, portrait.[7] For example, in 2022, white physicians comprised 69.2 percent of all clinical faculty positions, 79.6 percent of all full professor positions, and 81 percent of all department chair positions; Black physicians comprised 4.3 percent, 2.3 percent, 4 percent; Latinx physicians comprised 3.7 percent, 2.7 percent, 3.9 percent; and Asian physicians comprised 22.8 percent, 15.4 percent, 11.1 percent, respectively.[8] The AAMC does not publish comprehensive historical data on students' socioeconomic status, but in the AAMC Matriculating Student Questionnaire in 2016—which had a 50 percent response rate of the incoming cohort of U.S. medical students—of the 11,299 students who replied to the question about parental income, 33.3 percent of the students had a combined parental income of $200,000 and above, and an *additional* 32.3 percent of the students had a combined parental income of $100,000 and above.[9] Other research suggests that nearly a fifth of all current medical students have at least one parent who is a physician and, at every step of the medical school pipeline, students with more financial resources are at an advantage relative to their less-resourced peers.[10]

In this chapter, I examine the evolution of admissions criteria and curricular practices to foreground the relationship between the medical school and the reproduction of the profession in the United States. I show how medical schools have made—and continue to make—the profession. They do so individually as medical educators at each school train the next generation of physicians; they also do so collectively by interpreting profession-wide admissions and curricular standards, enacting these interpretations in the classroom, contributing to discussions about troubleshooting instruction, and competing with other schools to be leaders in the making of medical professionals. As I demonstrate in this chapter and throughout the book, what are inseparable from educators' conversations about *what it takes* to be a good physician are increasingly more implicit discussions about *which social groups* make good physicians. In other words, the professional identity of the physician is inextricable from the social identities of Jacobsen's—and others'—idealized well-rounded, white elite men.

U.S. MEDICINE AS A PROFESSIONALIZATION PROJECT

While there are many professions under the umbrella of health-care providers, medical doctors are both symbolically and politically dominant. Their power is both an historical and recurring achievement—in this sense, an ongoing professionalization project.[11] Before the turn of the twentieth century, those who practiced medicine in the U.S. medical field were marked by their heterogeneity, with an assortment of health-care practitioners peddling custom elixirs, small schools operating on an apprentice model, and sects of thought-leaders competing with one another.[12] Cohesion was elusive, and patient care was clinically limited.[13] As the profession organized to gain cultural authority and market power in the United Stares, the leaders adopted the Western European medical school form, characterized by the tripartite research-teaching-service model.[14] These leaders—and, by extension, the physicians training in these schools—simultaneously embraced, produced, and disseminated racist and misogynistic ideologies about patients and the social world.[15]

In addition to admissions protocols, curricular practices are a central vehicle for this reproduction of power. On the one hand, what medical students learn—whether formally or informally—has an impact on how they will eventually do their work and understand their roles as physicians. On the other hand, beyond the manifest function of teaching, curricular practices also reveal another core principle of U.S. medical education: teaching is a mechanism for profession-wide gatekeeping. Curricular practices, through their substantive and symbolic dimensions, thus play a pivotal role in how the profession upholds power. The decisions the medical profession made, historically (and contemporarily), about whether to recruit students with specific educational pedigrees or to teach them particular lessons from disparate disciplines reveal not only what the profession values but also who they value.

HUMANITIES AS PEDIGREE

Momentum was already underway for medical schools to tighten their admissions and curricular practices to gain legitimacy in the eyes of the U.S. government and public when the infamous Flexner report hit the newsstands. Published in 1910 by Abraham Flexner with funding from the Carnegie Foundation, this report expedited medical school leaders' restructuring processes.[16] In the wake of the report, medical students needed to possess a bachelor of arts or sciences degree to gain admission to an accredited medical school. They also needed to learn basic and clinical sciences, engage in hands-on training, and conduct research. Substantive knowledge and skills therefore became fundamental building blocks of the profession.[17] But so did credentials—that is, the status those bachelor's degrees represented.[18]

To elaborate further, before the Flexner-era professional consolidation in the first half of the twentieth century, physicians were not automatically regarded with high esteem nor were they compensated handsomely. Given the contemporary reputation of the humanities and social sciences relative to science, technology, engineering, mathematics, and medicine (STEMM) fields, it may seem ironic that part of the medical profession leaders' strategy in legitimizing medicine in the first half of the twentieth century was to incorporate the humanities so that physicians could be associated with a more prestigious profession: that of the academy.[19] Regarding the impact of the Flexner report, one medical educator opined in the flagship journal of the time, "soon a professor in clinical medicine became as respectable as a professor of classic literature at Harvard."[20] As historian Kenneth Ludmerer documented, citing the Flexner report, the leadership of the profession "wanted the requirement for admission to be a college degree because the popular stereotypes of 'coarse and common doctors' could be readily combated if *only cultivated persons* were permitted to become physicians" (emphasis added).[21]

Sociologist LaTonya Trotter has argued that it was precisely the cultural authority embodied by white elite men with which the leaders of the medical profession aligned themselves with when they had limited "curative" authority.[22] As the interdisciplinary scholar Moya Bailey aptly puts it, "Northern wealthy white men implicitly became the prototypical student as previous practices that served a more diverse student body were shed."[23] While Meharry Medical College, an historically Black college, was one of the thirty-one schools that did not need to close after Flexner released his findings, most medical schools training women and people of color closed after being unable to meet the new, post-Flexnerian standards for admissions and curricular practices.

Warren Weaver's address given to leaders of medical education at the AAMC annual meeting is emblematic of the profession's desire for admitting and training "only cultivated persons." Weaver was a philosopher and legal scholar who worked at the Alfred Sloan Foundation and the Rockefeller Foundation, two philanthropic organizations involved in funding the restructuring of medical schools during this post-Flexner, professional consolidation period. In his AAMC address introducing his friend, Dr. Alan Gregg, who was receiving an award for his work, Weaver further articulated the profile, or pedigree, of the ideal physician:[24]

> There are several aspects of his character on which I wish to comment. The first is his interest in words and in writing. When he was a student at Harvard he wrote verse for the *Advocate*, and in his senior year, was editor of the *Lampoon*. His literary friends urged him to go into writing as a career; and the elegance of style, richness and precision of language, and fascinating content of the many essays and lectures which he produced, during his scientific career are ample evidence that he could have starred as a professional writer. He was very gifted in languages, and, in success, he mastered French, Portuguese, German, and Italian. He had an insatiable appetite for and delight in the right word.[24]

I quote this at length to show just how much the humanities were celebrated for their character-producing qualities. From the 1920s through the 1960s, medical school leaders touted that their schools were in the "hands of devoted, public spirited men" who espoused "eternal values for society," "the will to be a leader," "excellence in character," and "flexible minds," and operated as a "technician as well as philosopher . . . poet as well as statistician," and looked "upon a patient as a 'whole human being.'"[25]

This professional adulation of the humanities was not merely lip service. Leaders of the medical profession acted on this sentiment of wanting cultivated students by creating an "Understanding Modern Society" section on the MCAT in 1946.[26] With these admissions standards, the humanities served as a proxy for pedigree. In other words, the profession's appreciation of the humanities as they consolidated in the early twentieth century was just as much oriented around who was going into medicine as it was about what a humanistic education could achieve in terms of knowledge, attitudes, and skills. For the latter, humanism and equity were described at this time as important values for grounding the profession's self-concept. As one medical educator noted at the 1953 AAMC annual meeting, "current interest in the teaching of the social and environmental factors in the undergraduate medical curriculum can be traced directly to a basic humanistic approach—that concern for all the health needs of human beings, which as always characterized the true physician."[27]

During a 1960 AAMC meeting, another medical educator argued for including the humanities for their critical and reflective capacities, saying:

What do we want the doctor and man to be like? I shall try a list: the ability to reason critically and to reach sound, i.e., testable judgments on one's own; knowledge enough to be able to start thinking in various areas of experience and types of situation and to know what should be known as grounds for judgment; curiosity and imagination, to project one's thought into the unfamiliar to discover the new; sensitivity and sensibility, the sort of feeling that supports the imagination in understanding people and situations and in aesthetic appreciation; social attitudes and criteria of decision and of behavior based on a considered non-egoistic value-structure.[28]

When it came to humanities content in the curricular practices of medical schools, by the 1930s, University of California, San Francisco (UCSF) and Johns Hopkins had departments of medical history within their medical schools, and forty-six of the accredited seventy-seven medical schools contained curriculum on medical history in 1939.[29] In less frequent cases, there were courses on philosophy, like one at a medical school in the 1950s that taught its students how to analyze "the theoretical premises of medicine in terms of ontology."[30]

While there was some coursework, the humanities were incorporated mostly before medical students matriculated into medical school. I call this the *inclusion-as-admissions* approach. With the inclusion-as-admissions approach, it is difficult to disentangle the social identity (e.g., white, elite, male) of the applicants and matriculants from the professional identity (e.g., soon-to-be physicians). Scholars engaged in the historical and contemporary work on the social reproduction of privilege have shown how the construction of "merit" often serves to maintain elites in power: from educational attainment to employment, merit is in the eye of the gatekeeping beholder, where "the definition of 'merit' is fluid and tends to reflect the values and interests of those in power to impose their particular cultural ideals."[31]

Just as employers used and interpreted various signals from a résumé to identify candidates with the right "fit," hoping to hire people like them, in what sociologist Lauren Rivera calls "looking glass merit," Carlyle Jacobsen and his 1949 looking glass vision of what constituted a good physician remains.[32] As "status displays," the contents of a résumé help students showcase their well-roundedness, and there are many opportunities for (pre)medical students to engage in status displays—not being a "dullard" is an important example of that. Valuing the humanities as a proxy for social pedigree is part of a subtle machinery that reproduces the professional status quo by reproducing what and who contains "meritorious" status. Vestiges of this inclusion-as-admissions approach remain with twenty-first-century undergraduate medical education (UME) practices, but the appreciation of the humanities started to fade in UME as the status of biomedical knowledge rose in the mid- to late twentieth century.

BIOMEDICAL AND PROFESSIONAL EXPANSION

The professional and cultural authority of the U.S. medical profession crystallized beginning in the mid-twentieth century. Physicians began enjoying what was termed the Golden Age of Doctoring, where their autonomy and power as health-care providers was perceived to be at its zenith. Scientific advances (e.g., germ theory, antibiotics), diagnostic technology (e.g., x-ray, stethoscope, blood tests), and specialization (e.g., expanded knowledge base, interdependence) all contributed to unifying the profession and bolstering the curative authority of its members.[33] The need for the explicit cultural authority captured in the humanities pedigree melted away as the promise of—and professional authority encapsulated in—biomedical science took hold. From the perspective of sociologists and medical professionals alike at this time, this alignment with biomedical science in the bio-bio-bio era seemed to absolve the profession of its white, Eurocentric, and paternalistic roots.[34]

If the post-Flexner era was oriented around the standardization of education in a research-teaching-service model, the post–Golden Age was oriented around the growth of biomedical research and clinical practice at the expense of focusing on teaching medical students.[35] The rise of the promise of technoscientific biomedicine was accompanied by a concomitant expansion in the number of basic and clinical faculty, the growth of the academic medical center, the increase in public and private research funding for biomedicine, and the proliferation of health care services in general. In the 1930s, the power to decide the direction of the medical school was consolidated with the university president, but by the 1970s, there was a large-scale administrative and bureaucratic infrastructure with the expansion of deans, course directors, offices, and departments within the medical school.[36] Clinical faculty members were installed as the central decision makers and implementers of curricular design and facilitation.

This rapid biomedicalization in the mid- to late twentieth century also increased the amount of biomedical knowledge that physicians could and should know.[37] The medical school entrance requirements changed in favor of more biomedical sciences and clinical experience and less humanities and social sciences.[38] In the central journal of the profession, *Academic Medicine*, the very little material on history began taking on a triumphalist bent, with biographies celebrating the great (white) men and their biomedical achievements. In these biographies, there was no sociohistorical contextualization about how— and at whose expense—these biomedical discoveries were achieved. Similarly, by 1969, only thirty-three of eighty-five medical schools included history in their UME curricular practices, which is just thirty-nine percent of schools compared to the sixty percent a few decades prior. Medical school leaders were no longer looking explicitly for "well-rounded" white elite men; they were looking for biomedical scientists.

A group of reformers organized in the 1960s around the emerging discipline of "medical humanities," an approach combining methodologies from history, philosophy, literature, and the arts, to produce insights on the "art of medicine."[39] In 1969, a group of physicians and humanities scholars formed the Society for Health and Human Values (SHHV) to encourage a more thoughtful and widespread inclusion of the humanities into medical education. With funding from the National Endowment for the Humanities (NEH), this group had expansive discussions around the role of the physician in addressing inequalities, the progressing encroachment of the biomedical sciences over other forms of humanistic and interpretive knowledge, and the ethical considerations accompanying the emerging new clinical and research technologies.[40] Their attempts at systematically incorporating critical humanities content into UME curricular practices mostly failed; any lingering humanities content was folded into bioethics programs, which are notoriously "thin" with regard to substance and individualistic with regard to focus.[41]

A familiarity or fluency with humanities (or social sciences) was no longer deemed essential for American physicians, signaled by the removal of this content—which had been captured in the "Understanding Modern Society" section—from the MCAT in 1977.[42] Fewer medical school initiates held degrees in humanities and social sciences fields (and there were fewer of these majors from the cohort of college graduates in general).[43] In 1979, the budget for the National Science Foundation (NSF) was five times that of the NEH, but by 1997, it was thirty times as much—and only 0.45 percent of the federal research support budget went to the humanities in 2010.[44] The medical professional and broader academic landscape was changing in favor of scientific research, and while the bulk of that favor went to biomedical science, social science also benefitted.

THE ENTRANCE OF THE POSITIVISTIC AND PATERNALISTIC SOCIAL SCIENCES

Swept up in the medical profession's overarching investment in science, interest in the social sciences proliferated at AAMC annual meetings. At the 1960 meeting, for example, leaders discussed how medical schools must build programs to capitalize on the rapidly increasing financial support for medical research—public dollars alone were $45 million in 1940 and $330 million in 1957—suggesting that they build up around new disciplines such as medical genetics and atomic medicine *as well as* psychology, sociology, and anthropology in the medical school faculties, curriculum, and research programs.[45] The resulting "behavioral health movement" in medical education entailed social scientists attempting to integrate their knowledge into medical education in the 1960s, with the help of funding from the National Institute of Child Health and Development (NICHD) and National Institute of Mental Health (NIMH).

With these nationally sponsored and profession-wide reports, the medical educators articulated an aspirational position about integrating the social sciences as part of the fundamental building blocks of medical education, which is more of an *inclusion-as-integration* approach. Less about who, in terms of pedigree, was being admitted, these early social sciences inclusion attempts were more about essential skills and knowledge—but these essential skills and knowledge were *not* steeped in a critical tradition.[46] An example of the inclusion-as-integration approach can be found in the proceedings from a 1970 NICHD meeting on the "Behavioral Sciences in Medical Education." In the published proceedings, the interdisciplinary group of social science scholars and clinical faculty members enumerated the ways in which the behavioral and social sciences would be important for clinical practice:

- theoretical knowledge about human behavior;
- make students aware that the patient is a human being with a family, with feelings, with problems, and with a job;
- look both at social factors as variables in disease processes and at the effect of disease processes on social structure and behavior;
- illuminate processes involved in patient/professional interrelationships;
- cast light on decision-making processes in health care;
- identify social and cultural changes involved in technological development and innovations in medical practice;
- and shed light on the social and cultural values, norms, and ideologies of medical schools.[47]

What is notable about these social scientific lessons here is that they were markedly uncritical of the medical profession and its legacies in perpetuating harm to marginalized groups.

In the *Academic Medicine* journal there were rejoinders regarding the "obvious" need for the understanding of more structural social science material, like studying "urbanization, industrialization, change in value systems, secularization."[48] But those rejoinders were glaringly silent about racism, patriarchy, and capitalism. Those rejoinders were also largely drowned out by the profession actively engaging in exclusionary political practices and by medical educators emphasizing more positivistic and paternalistic social science. Through curricular and gatekeeping practices—even ones that seemed aimed at encouraging humane and equitable health care with the inclusion-as-integration approach—the U.S. medical profession reinforced the vision of a physician as a white, elite expert and the patient as the nonwhite, nonelite, uninformed Other.

Regarding the exclusionary political practices, movements—for example, the women's health movement and the Black Panther Party's People's Free Medical Clinics—that provided curricular programming for physicians that included critiques of classist, sexist, heteronormative, and racist practices within U.S. health care were notably *external* to the medical profession.[49] While a small minority of physicians participated in these movements, they were individual exceptions to what was otherwise a socially and fiscally conservative professional rule.[50] In addition to mounting a lobby to block the creation of Medicaid and Medicare and continuing to ration admissions spots in medical schools to maintain the market power of physicians, the professionally dominant American Medical Association (AMA) did not support Black physicians during the civil rights movement, instead deferring to the state-level racist practices excluding Black physicians from membership.[51] Therefore, over the course of the latter half of the twentieth century, the U.S. medical profession politically acted—whether actively or passively—to continue reinforcing the white elite social identity of the profession.

With regard to the medical profession's embrace of positivistic social sciences, or the pursuit of "objective facts" about social groups through mostly quantitative methods, in *Academic Medicine* there was an uptick in discussions of psychological tests utilized by admissions committees, which reflected an overall shift from a focus on "character" to a focus on "characteristics."[52] While the prior research has emphasized how admissions committees have become enamored with the "objectivity" that positivistic social science seemed to promise—as well as the shift in focus to student performance over substance—this work has overlooked what comprised that "character" to begin with. The use of psychological tests to observe characteristics also reflects the start of U.S. professions drawing on a body of knowledge that rhetorically shifted the responsibility of, say, institutional racism to the implicit, cognitive biases of physicians, absolving the profession of blame.[53]

With support from the federal government, statistics-heavy social scientific research on health disparities also took off during the latter half of the twentieth century.[54] In 1999, Congress solicited a study from the Institute of Medicine (IOM) to assess the significant racial and ethnic disparities in health and health care, as reported in the landmark report *Unequal Treatment*. The report was accompanied by the Minority Health and Health Disparities Research and Education Act of 2000, which amended Public Law 106–525 and was aimed at improving the health of socially marginalized patients.[55] This act established the creation of admissions protocols for underrepresented students at medical schools, loan repayment by the federal government for minority health research, the installment of centers for health disparities research in numerous universities in the United States, and the establishment of an evaluation and reporting mechanism for the Agency on Healthcare Research and Quality (AHRQ).[56]

As positivistic social science was on the rise, so, too, was paternalistic social science. The paternalistic social science that oozed into medical education at this time emanated from cultural anthropological approaches to patients. Patients—particularly nonwhite and poor ones—were conceptualized as "the primitive Other" to be objectively observed and known, and this paternalistic approach was embodied in cultural competence curricular practices. When medical schools adopted "competencies," like the Liaison Committee on Medical Education's (LCME) "universal competencies," one of them was cultural competence, which became required by medical school accreditation boards in 2000.[57] At its best, cultural competence encouraged the creation of empathic clinicians with the capacity to take the lived experiences of patients into consideration for diagnosis and treatment. At its worst, as many scholars have noted, it led to clinicians exoticizing the nonwhite, nonheteronormative, non-American Other and denying the examination of Western biomedicine itself as a culture.[58]

With the entrance of the social sciences, there may have been more substantive goals in the inclusion-as-integration approach to incorporating these topics into curricular practices, but the social scientists came from the same white, elite, and paternalistic social position as the humanists and clinicians. Thus, even though the ideal clinician was constructed as holding humanistic values and marshalling interpretive tools from the social sciences, most of the social science that was incorporated or embraced served to uphold white elite paternalism—just like the way that the humanities embodied a distinct pedigree. The paternalism—that the clinician can know better—thus relied on multiple disciplines that valued knowledge collected in a specific kind of way (e.g., positivist, imperialist).

CURRICULAR PRACTICES AND PROFESSIONAL POWER

I give this history of the humanities and social sciences in U.S. medical education over the course of the twentieth century not only to contextualize the contemporary inclusion of these fields but also to confound the rosy, romantic narrative of the promise of these disciplines. Curricular practices reflect what physicians confront, what they perceive to be important, and who is an authority about what needs to be known—the physicians relative to the patients, experts relative to laypeople, the rich relative to the poor, the white person relative to the person of color, the biomedical knowledge relative to the humanistic and social scientific knowledge. To understand further how the social sciences and humanities are incorporated in the twenty-first century, I must set up how I am conceptualizing curricular practices and how they reproduce the medical profession.

Produced during the Golden Age of Doctoring, with physicians at the height of their autonomy, the foundational sociological texts about the medical profession, *The Student Physician* and *Boys in White*, focused on the value formation and socialization processes that shaped future physicians.[59] These studies were largely uncritical of the medical profession, its relationship to patients, and the structure of the healthcare system.[60] Further work on the profession focused on the technical knowledge that physicians held jurisdiction over, without questioning the political implications of that knowledge itself.[61] These foundational arguments by sociologists provided insight into some of the ways that curricular practices operated, but tended to depict medical socialization and professionalization processes as apolitical.

In another subfield, sociologists in education have posed the concepts of formal, informal, hidden, and null curricula to elucidate different conceptualizations of curricular outcomes. In general, the requirements that medical students must meet to receive their medical degree are contained in the *formal curriculum*, or the deliberately designed materials and coursework. The curricular maps and course descriptions I draw on are exemplative in this regard. In contrast to what is explicit is the *informal curriculum*, which captures the indirect instruction that is facilitated by educators' and peers' actions, as well as the *hidden curriculum*, which illustrates the disconnect between what students are taught and what students learn. Although the concept of the hidden curriculum has been used as an analytical tool with differing definitions, the original usage of the concept draws attention to how the hidden curriculum inheres in the medical school's spatial and technological infrastructure, distribution of power, policies, evaluative standards, allocated resources, and institutional slang.[62] Finally, the *null curriculum*, while notoriously ambiguous, has been used to describe what is excluded from curricular practices.[63]

I find these discussions of types of curriculum to be too focused on outcomes rather than the process with which educators make decisions that create these outcomes in the first place. I anchor my analysis with a focus on *curricular practices* to show how faculty members actively and dynamically shape students. More important, I focus on how curricular practices are productive and ideological. They are *productive* because they denote actions, or enactments of design and implementation, that occur from matriculation to graduation. They are *ideological* because they denote the conceptualizations of the relationships between profession and school, faculty members and students, biomedicine and the humanities and social sciences, physicians and patients. Taken together, as a site of potential and continuous change, curricular practices are consequential because they constitute the quotidian and agenda-setting ways in which a medical school— and thus the medical profession—reproduces itself and the attendant inhumanities and inequalities that come with it.

Students have many sources of knowledge about how to become— and what it means to be—a physician, from the classroom (lectures, small groups, standardized patient exercises) to the clinic (patients, experiences, lab results), to research (laboratory techniques, collaborators), to the community (other professions, community members).[64] Given all these sources of socialization, in conceptualizing curricular practices as productive, I am drawing attention to how medical educators—at the profession-wide and individual medical school level—are engaged in social practices that organize and distribute knowledge. Curricular practices are "modes of working and doing."[65] Thinking of curricular practices as productive social practices orients us to sets of action that are shaped by the cultural and organizational context but are ultimately enacted by actors.

Another benefit to thinking of curricular practices as productive is that it focuses attention on how curricular practices constitute a nested set of pragmatic decisions made at different levels of analysis and thus reveals the dynamic process of knowledge application. First, there is the bird's-eye view of curricular dreams and policies at the level of the profession. Leaders in the medical profession design standards for what students are to learn and when. Second, these same big-picture decisions are made at the level of the individual medical school, where medical educators deliberate how to enact the programming suggested and standards required by the professional governing bodies. Practically speaking, curricular practices express power through this very agenda-setting capacity. Third, medical educators are engaged in active production through their mundane, everyday implementation of curricular practices. While a culmination of a series of nested decisions, it is through these curricular practices that medical students receive instruction—this is how they are finally made into physicians.

In viewing the parts of this process together, curricular practices—in the medical profession leaders' and school-based educators' toggling between conceptualizing standards and implementing them—thus comprise the pragmatic mechanism by which the profession maintains its power. Curricular practices can always be updated and that flexibility breeds power.[66] Each curricular reform is an opportunity for the profession to identify, react to, and absorb critique; each curricular reform is an opportunity for the profession to reassert its power. Similarly, each curricular standard is an opportunity for a medical school to interpret as it sees fit; each curricular standard is an opportunity for a medical school to make its mark.

Curricular practices are thus also ideological. Not only are curricular practices an outcome of collective action, hence political; they are also a profession's articulation of a vision of the social world. They are the connective tissue between educators, students, schools, the profession, patients, and knowledge, articulating what the relationships between these various groups *should* look like. Curricular practices posit formal roles (e.g., instructor, student) and set the conditions for informal roles to arise (e.g., mentor, mentee)—providing a window into the way relationships operate in a medical school. Most crucially here, however, is *who* these educators and students are. As the history of UME suggests, the concern with including an appreciation of the humanities and social sciences is not new, and it has always been linked with the larger professional project where the image of the good physician was one of a distinct social identity. As legal scholar Leah Goodridge has argued, "professionalism" is thinly veiled white and elite and male cultural capital.[67] Historically, these (mostly male) students came from white and elite families, and they also rewarded their cultural capital, in turn folding into the conceptualization of the profession a distinctly white, distinctly elitist, and distinctly masculine set of values.[68] These values remain in curricular practices in the early twenty-first century, even if they are less explicit.

* * *

What does the history of curricular practices, particularly for social scientific and humanistic knowledge, tell us? It tells us a few important components about what a profession values, who it values, and how the profession reproduces itself. First, these characteristics indicate an historical appreciation for the humanities—that the humanities assist in cultivating a physician with an admirable pedigree—one who is "well rounded." Second, they also show an appreciation of the social sciences, particularly of the positivistic and paternalistic variety, rather than that of structural and critical perspectives. Third, these forms of appreciation reek of white, elite, male entitlement. The central difference between the curricular injustices then versus now is that there are now more possibilities for critical and reflective engagement—but those perspectives are still rarely the ones being included.[69]

2

PROFESSION-WIDE CURRICULAR DREAMS

D r. Walcker, a white woman, embodied a prototypical clinical faculty member at a U.S. academic medical center in 2015. She saw patients in the clinic, led a team of residents on rotations, taught in the medical school's clinical skills course, participated on curriculum committees, and tried to find the time with all that to stay on top of all her administrative work *and* up to date on the latest clinical guidelines. It was a harried daily existence, but Dr. Walcker believed in the academic medicine model that combined clinical work, student instruction, and research. She wanted to engage in the best possible clinical practices and help future physicians do the same.

One thing she noticed in her decades of experience in these roles was that the profession was in dire need of curricular change. As she explained to me,

> One of the reasons students come into medicine is because these are highly idealistic individuals who are going to work hard. They want to help others, and they want to see the world change. We traditionally have not given them the tools to teach them how to change the world. These kids do not want to feel disempowered, they do not want to feel cynical, they do not want to feel disenchanted and discouraged. But something we've been doing in medical education for decades makes them feel that way most of the time.

Walcker was not alone in expressing these sentiments. Many medical educators—especially those with clinical backgrounds—with whom I spoke during my research on curricular practices in contemporary U.S. medical education frequently told me how essential it was for them to imbue medical education with humanity, meaning, and a greater understanding of social experiences and inequalities.

After telling me about the disempowerment, disenchantment, and discouragement that medical students confront, Walcker continued by pointing to the humanities as holding the "tools" to help students feel differently. Indeed, the clinical faculty members I interviewed and the broader professional governing bodies, like the Association of American Medical Colleges (AAMC), invoked the humanities and social sciences as solutions to different problems plaguing medical education and clinical practice.

If the cognitive jump from Walcker's construction of the problems—for example, "they want to help others" and "they do not want to feel disenchanted"—to her invocation of the humanities as a solution seems to be missing some key connections, it does. Through the course of my research, the clinical faculty members' pathways from problem to solution often lacked clarity, and their conceptualization of the humanities and social sciences varied in substance and complexity. Scholars of medical education, through their individual case studies of particular schools and their scoping reviews, have also drawn attention to the heterogenous and inconsistent ways in which medical educators have conceptualized the humanities and social sciences.[1] Generally, the humanities contain disciplines such as literature, art, philosophy, and history, and while disciplinary differences abound, the field is oriented around the close and critical inquiry of human expression and experience. The social sciences encapsulate disciplines such as anthropology, sociology, and economics, and while this field also has important disciplinary distinctions, it is dedicated to describing and explaining human behaviors, relationships, and systems.

In this chapter, I unpack how the profession proposed the humanities and social sciences as solutions to various problems in the early twenty-first-century, focusing on how medical educators constructed their curricular dreams and illustrating their trajectories into programming and standards. I call them curricular dreams because dreaming is often vague and varied, and, of course, it can be just that: dreaming. Undergraduate medical education (UME) is often where many clinical faculty members, like Walcker, engaged in the "infusion"—to quote another respondent of mine, white male clinical faculty member Dr. Bernansky—of the humanities and social sciences. To help set the stage for where educators pitch these curricular dreams, I start by describing the basic curricular structure of most medical schools in the United States. Then I detail the medical educators' different constructions of *why* they think the humanities and social sciences are needed and *what* they want to include from the humanities and social sciences for training future physicians. I end the chapter with the programming and standards that the medical profession had established as recommendations for the humanities, and requirements for the social sciences, within UME.

SITUATING CURRICULAR PRACTICES IN UNDERGRADUATE MEDICAL EDUCATION

Medical school is hard, like really hard. Of course, the road to becoming a physician starts far before a student matriculates into medical school for their UME.[2] Students must earn exceptional grades, particularly in the basic and biomedical sciences. Students must gain exposure to health professions by shadowing in a clinic or volunteering in a hospital. Students must be familiar with scientific research and take on leadership positions in organizations. Before matriculating into medical school, students must compete for a limited spot in a competitive profession.[3] While it has grown over time, the medical profession has not kept pace with the growing patient population; in 1961, there were eighty-six medical schools and 6,994 medical school graduates (with 180 million people in the United States); by 1981, there were 126 schools and 15,985 graduates (with 226 million people.); by 2018, there were 137 schools and 19,553 graduates (with 326 million people).[4]

When medical students matriculate into a U.S. medical school to undergo the four years of UME, they are beginning the next phase of a multiple-step process to becoming a physician who will practice without direct supervision. The purpose of UME is to provide students with the foundational theoretical knowledge and practical skills that will prove to be the pillars of their future clinical practice. After all, curricular practices are productive; at the end of the UME, they produce physicians, as symbolized by their medical doctor (MD) degree. Accredited medical schools have roughly the same curricular structure, where students engage in preclinical coursework for the first eighteen to twenty-four months and then participate in approximately a year of clinical rotations or clerkships; in the final year, they hit the interview trail for residency programs while they round out their training with various electives (see figure 2.1 for a visual representation of this structure).

During preclinical coursework, medical educators teach the foundational theoretical knowledge and begin modeling the skills and attitudes for clinical practice. The theoretical knowledge constituting this coursework is dominated by the basic and clinical sciences, as captured by a representative description from one medical school:

> This course surveys principles of genetics, and molecular, cellular and developmental biology in relation to human disease processes. Coverage includes basics of cell cycle regulation, gene expression, protein processing, signal transduction, ion transport and action potentials, genetics, embryology, cancer biology, immunology and pharmacology. Laboratory sessions provide an overview of cell structure and tissue organization along with thematically relevant concepts of histopathology.

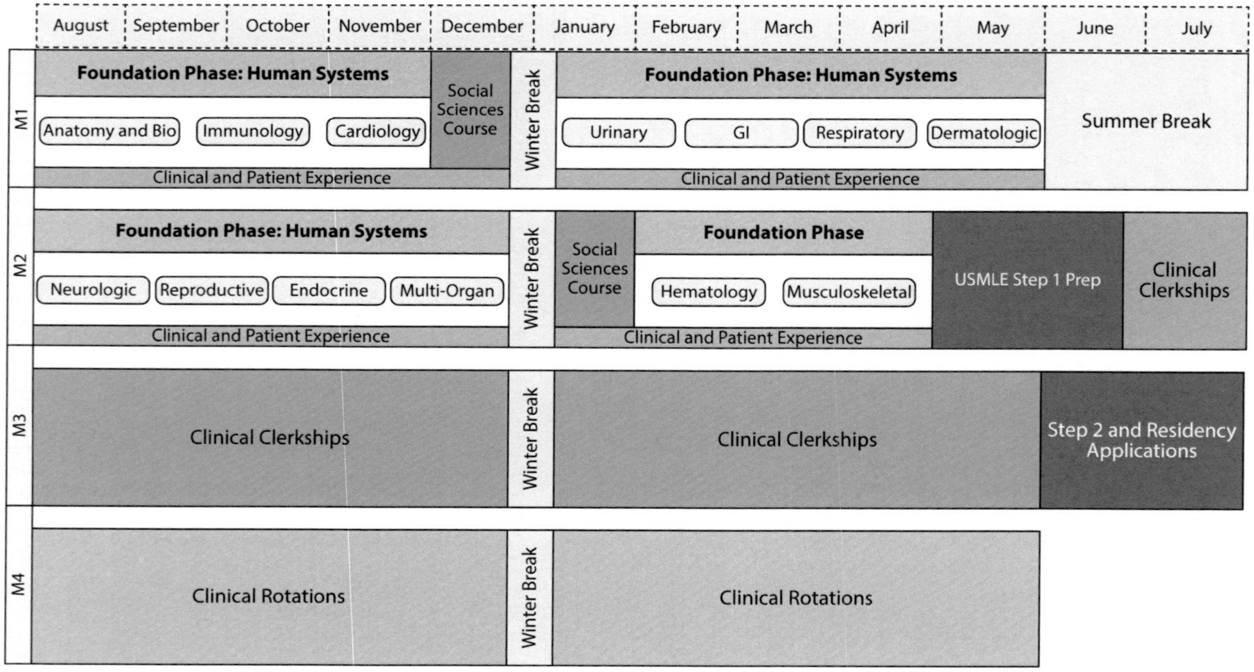

FIGURE 2.1 Preclinical curriculum schematic

Courses like this are largely taught by basic scientists or clinical faculty whose expertise is in one of these particular areas. These core courses denote a scientific model for approaching medicine, with course titles such as "Genes to Cells". They also take up a significant portion of the first part of the preclinical phase, as evident in figure 2.1. As another example, in a sixteen-week "Molecules to Cells and Tissues" course at another medical school, students gained "knowledge of fundamental concepts in molecular, cell and tissue biology and in clinical genetics," which would then "enable them to explain the molecular, biochemical and cellular underpinnings of health and various disease states."

After mastering the foundational theoretical knowledge, students generally integrate this knowledge into the next topic: organ systems. Students cover organ systems in blocks, and these courses are also taught by both basic and clinical faculty. As one school detailed, they go through: "the musculoskeletal system; cancer biology; the neuro-logic system; the cardiovascular and pulmonary systems; the renal, endocrine, gastrointestinal, and reproductive systems; immunology, microbiology, hematology, rheumatology, dermatology; nephrology, pulmonary disease, cardiology, gastroenterology; neurology, psychiatry, endocrinology, men's and women's health." With each of these blocks, students are taught through lecture and are tested on their knowledge with frequent exams.

In addition to the foundational knowledge usually taught in the context of a lecture and organized by block, all medical students engage in a course where they learn the practical skills of "doctoring." While I will describe this course in further detail in chapter 3 and 4, for the sake of this brief overview, it is important to know that this course is usually facilitated by clinical faculty members, and (in more rare cases) by a combination of clinical faculty members and other health-care professionals (e.g., nurses, occupational therapists, or social workers) or scholars from other disciplines (e.g., social science and humanities). While this course may be called something different depending on the individual school, a common name for it is the

"Practice of Medicine" (POM). One school describes their version of a POM course as one that:

> covers a wide range of essential topics related to the practice of medicine such as professionalism, leadership, ethics, patient safety, health policy, health care law, research design, epidemiology, and more. It is a longitudinal curriculum that runs across all four years of the curriculum. [POM] gives you the opportunity to learn and practice skills physicians use every day including communication and interpersonal skills, teamwork, history taking, physical examination, and simple procedures. You begin applying these skills in our virtual clinic with standardized patients and in our virtual hospital with high-fidelity patient simulators. You work closely with the coaching of Scholar-Advisors in a low-stress environment to prepare you to succeed in the real clinical environment.

As this course description suggests, when students are in the POM doctoring courses, they learn through a few modalities: lecture, small-group discussions, panels, and standardized patient encounters. In figure 2.1, the POM sequence is called "Clinical and Patient Experience," and it is longitudinally threaded throughout the majority of the first two years of UME.

As I will show in subsequent chapters, most medical educators include the social sciences within the first two years of preclinical curriculum, whether in a course or in the POM sequence. They tend to include the humanities in either the first two years or the final year as an elective. In figure 2.1, for example, students would receive the social sciences during their "Social Sciences" course but the humanities would not materialize on the curricular map. In rare cases that I will describe in the conclusion to this book, medical educators would have a separate block or a separate longitudinal thread that includes social sciences or humanities content.

Medical educators place a high value on clinical experience, so much so that at many medical schools, the preclinical curriculum has been reduced (from twenty-four to eighteen months) so that students can get to their clerkships in their second year. The third year of UME is dedicated to clinical rotations, when students move from specialty to specialty. When students finish rotations, they then have opportunities to take more electives. The fourth year can be highly individualized as medical students vie for residency positions; therefore, there is less required coursework that would be common to all students at this time in their training. The electives students take in their last year tend to be either research-intensive or extra rotations within a particular specialty so they can put themselves in the best possible position for their coveted program for residency.

While getting into medical school is difficult and doing well in the coursework is important, one of the major professional pressures for medical students is the step 1 portion of the United States Medical Licensing Exam (USMLE). Students need to do well on it so they can have a good shot at a desirable residency, although other scholars have shown that a high step 1 score does not guarantee an admission into a top residency program because the prestige of the UME program also matters a tremendous amount.[5] After students complete the UME and receive their MD degree, they will matriculate into residency programs, where they will receive additional training in their chosen specialty. After training in their specialty, they may elect to undergo more specialized training in the form of a fellowship, or they may begin practicing as a fully trained physician.

As evident in this description of the process by which a student matriculates into and then graduates from UME, there is a fair amount of potential for variation in the basic structure of curricular practices. In addition, these curricular practices are a site of much consternation—as Dr. Walcker described in the opening of this chapter: "something we've been doing in medical education for decades" was awry and in need of change. In many ways, the annual national meeting for medical educators held by the AAMC is oriented around and convened to troubleshoot curricular practices and thus improve the profession. The AAMC annual meetings are sites where many curricular dreams are articulated, workshopped, and critiqued. I will now turn my attention to the profession-wide discursive constructions of curricular practices and why medical educators evoke the humanities and social sciences as necessary for the future of the profession.

CLINICALLY RELEVANT PROBLEMS

Walcker's account underscored a sentiment that many clinical faculty members shared with me about what was wrong with UME. When I conducted my interviews with medical educators, after I asked them whether they taught any humanities or social sciences, I would ask them why. Even though there were several respondents that pointed to external pressures, which I will describe in a later section, the clinical faculty members would invariably point to the internal problems they felt that these fields could address. These problems largely fall under the umbrellas of *equity problems* or *empathy problems*. Equity problems concern the social inequalities affecting health, the provision of health care, and the physician workforce, whereas empathy problems entail patient (dis)satisfaction and physician burnout. In my interviews and in professional reports, the medical profession constructed many of these problems and their curricular solutions in the same breath, even if the connection was not entirely clear.

The medical profession was not the first—nor the only one—to illuminate these equity and empathy problems, but their voices were the loudest at the curricular dreaming phase. If the Flexner report was the professional game changer of the twentieth century for the U.S. medical profession, the 2003 Institute of Medicine (IOM) report on health and health-care inequalities was the watershed moment for the twenty-first century. The report was damning, albeit for different reasons than those of the Flexner report.[6] Not only did the IOM report show how the patient population was suffering, but it also noted that physicians, unfortunately, were part of the problem. As a result, the U.S. government backed the authors' policy recommendations, demanding that social inequalities be addressed by the medical profession; perhaps this was because latest estimates posit that these inequalities cost the United States hundreds of billions of dollars annually.[7] Medical students, too—whether individually or in certain groups, like the White Coats for Black Lives group—also called for more attention to social inequalities within the curricular practices of medical schools.[8]

Many of the clinical faculty members I spoke to felt deeply committed to ameliorating the equity problem. Take Dr. Li, an Asian male clinical faculty member and director of UME curriculum at his medical school. He told me his story about how he got involved in medical education. He started by saying, "[I]n medical school, you know, I'm learning the basic sciences, the same things as everybody else. Then clinical sciences, but I kept *seeing* at the time—I mean I wasn't as nuanced in my perspective as I am now—but I kept *seeing* health disparity after health disparity in the field and I didn't understand how we were not talking about any of that." In the clinic, he was seeing these social inequalities—what I call *clinical witnessing*—but the curricular practices he was experiencing did not do anything to address them. Li concluded, saying, "It was just horrific to me. I was like, 'We're just going to pretend that this is not happening?'" Representative of the current generation of clinical faculty who serve as medical educators, Li had no instruction on the social inequalities that he "kept seeing" in clinical settings.

There was a sense among the medical educators with whom I spoke that, while prior generations of physicians had ignored the social sciences and equity problems, that time was now over. Dr. Robinson, a white female clinical faculty member and dean of UME at another medical school, explained how this sentiment was turning, noting that "there have always been some people, who think that the touchy-feely stuff isn't important. But I think there [are] fewer of those folks than there used to be and I think that if you look at how people approach their education and practice of medicine, you'll see a lot more appreciation of the social role of healthcare and the social contributors." The clinical faculty members in my sample consistently expressed how they appreciated the need for addressing social inequalities. Their profession faced a significant equity problem, and their clinical witnessing helped them, quite literally, to see it.

Some social sciences and humanities faculty members also linked clinical faculty members' understanding of the equity problems to those faculty members' clinical experiences. For example, Dr. Pultz, a white female social scientist at one medical school, recounted, "I work with clinicians who are—for example, my chair is an endocrinologist and he studies diabetes." She continued, "[H]e's quite senior in the field and right now thinks that the biggest issue to contend with is poverty and social determinants of health." Pultz also said that, according to the experiences and considerations of this chair, he felt that "no matter how big of strides we've made with medicine related to diabetes, if we don't fix those structural and system issues, people will not be able to manage their disease in an optimal way." For Pultz's chair, his clinical witnessing of social inequalities drove his understanding of the equity problem.

A similar discourse about *empathy problems* emerged from my respondents and was mirrored in professional publications. At the end of the twentieth century, patients, as a countervailing power, wanted more empathy in the clinical encounter.[9] While patient needs are part of the empathy problem, clinical experiences steered a lot of the conceptualization of the empathy problem toward the physicians themselves. Within this understanding, physicians, who are increasingly governed by the market and bureaucratic logics that accompany U.S. health care, were experiencing more and more role strain and burnout. Of the ninety medical educators and students I interviewed at medical schools across the United States, fifty-six invoked the "problem of burnout" as a pressing issue, and they were overwhelmingly

MDs or in the MD pipeline. Burnout always came up in reference to including the humanities in curricular practices—and I did not have a single question about burnout, emotions, stress, or wellness in my interview guide.

Physician burnout and patient dissatisfaction were often discussed in the same breath for the clinical faculty members. Dr. George, a white male clinical faculty member, started describing the state of the profession by saying, "I do think that health care in America is at a time of crisis, and more and more people are writing about burnout, writing about dissatisfaction." He went on, "[A]nd it's not just a hot topic—it's real. *I feel it. I've felt it for years.* It's growing." After telling me about the acuity and personal palpability of the empathy problem, he continued with what he felt needed to change: "We need to infuse the medical space with meaning for the patient and for the health-care attendants, so I think it feels like we're doing meaningful work." For George, the lack of meaning for patients could transfer to physicians; empathy problems were mutually constitutive.

George's words also point to how clinical—and curricular—experiences inform the clinical faculty members' understanding of the importance of the empathy problem. Some of these issues with the current, biomedically heavy curricular practices were evoked by Dr. Schumann, a white female clinical faculty member, who said, "[Y]ou know, physicians have the highest rate of suicide because they've been taught everything is about science and medicine and so their humanity is in, some ways, just cut out of that." While Schumann pointed to the high stakes of burnout for physicians, another white female clinical faculty member, Dr. Johnson, articulated how burnout can also have an impact on patients, explaining how "burned-out clinicians are more likely to be rude to their patients. That's not good for anybody, and we don't want to lose clinicians to burnout or depression or alcohol abuse or whatever; and we also don't want them to mistreat patients in the middle of that." Thus, the empathy problem is clinically relevant for both physicians and patients. The stakes are high, too, because the burned-out physician is constructed as a source of potential patient harm—a consequential leap that the clinical faculty members did *not* make when discussing the equity problem.

Like Schumann and Johnson, my respondents' attention to these problems reflects a broader trend within the field of medical education. At the last several annual meetings of the AAMC, physician and student burnout and attendant material on student wellness constituted thematic threads for panels and presentations by and for medical educators. Often pitched as a national epidemic or burnout "crisis," medical students and educators were, at least discursively, concerned about the mental and physical livelihoods of members of their field—and for good reason. In 2014, the year before I started data collection, more than half of physicians surveyed in a national study reported that they were experiencing emotional exhaustion, loss of meaning in work, or a sense of ineffectiveness and lack of engagement with patients.[10]

At another AAMC meeting presentation on the humanities and arts in medical education, two presenters described how they led a comics elective where students were told to "tell a story that is meaningful to you." The educators—and audience, for that matter—were struck by how prevalent feelings of isolation, loneliness, and shame were in the comics that the medical students drew, and how often zombie and dehumanizing imagery were invoked. When I asked medical student Dylan, a white male medical student, what drew him to take an "Art and Medicine" elective, he replied, "I felt like I needed a break. I was going crazy." Chris, another white male medical student said, "[M]edical school's pretty stressful and [the humanities] can help us cope." With these examples, it shows how difficult it was to disentangle the problems with medical education and clinical practice from the humanities-as-curricular-solutions because the clinical faculty members and medical students would discuss them as a package.

In sum, in conversations, presentations, and publications, the medical profession conveyed that they were facing both equity and empathy problems. Of course, they were not the first nor only ones to draw attention to these problems, given that government, academic, patient, community, and student groups have been highlighting these problems for decades. And, of course, curricular solutions to these equity and empathy problems are just one slice of the solution pie. But what is important here is that the medical profession sought curricular solutions to these problems. And in reaching for curricular solutions, medical educators both enabled and constrained how the humanities and social sciences could be brought to bear on the improvement of medical education.

DREAMING ABOUT THE SOCIAL SCIENCES AND HUMANITIES AS CURRICULAR SOLUTIONS

For many medical educators, most of whom were clinical faculty members, the solutions to these equity and empathy problems came in the form of the social sciences and humanities, despite not really knowing much about these fields, a point I will return to in chapter 3. If all I had done was collect data at the annual meetings of the AAMC, I would have walked away with the notion that the medical profession was wild about addressing the inhumanities and inequities in patient care through curricular reform. Panels on the humanities were hot, and the participants were jazzed to be there; panels on the social sciences were packed, too, but with more head nodding and hand-wringing than buzzing enthusiasm.

At this curricular dreaming phase, clinical, social sciences, and humanities faculty members constructed many versions of the value of the humanities and social sciences, even though the clinical faculty members' voices were the most dominant. The social scientists and humanists who worked within the U.S. medical education field worked within their respective schools or in multischool partnerships to advance curricular solutions, but they were rarely organized. By way of quick contrast, in the United Kingdom, for example, social scientists organized and instigated the Todd report, leading to the incorporation of sociological training into medical education; in the United States, no such mobilization has occurred by professional bodies such as the American Sociological Association or the Modern Language Association.[11]

Clinical faculty members' main rationale undergirding the curricular promise of the humanities and social sciences is perhaps best captured by the words of the AAMC president, Darrell Kirch, as he introduced the new version of the MCAT in 2015:

> Being a good physician is about more than scientific knowledge. It is about understanding people—how they think, interact, and make decisions. Together with a solid foundation in the natural sciences, an understanding of behavior, perception, culture, poverty, and other concepts from psychology and sociology all contribute to the well-rounded physician. Of course, we want our doctors to understand how chemical compounds interact so our prescriptions do not have adverse interactions. But we also want our doctors to have good bedside manner, communication skills, and an ability to interact with people.[12]

Medical educators in my study also discussed curricular initiatives like that of the MCAT as part of a change occurring in the field oriented around the importance of "understanding humans."

With the educators' remarks and Kirch's press release, a few components stand out about the humanities and social sciences as curricular solutions put forth by the medical profession. First, curricular solutions are within the profession's control. Control over the content and direction of their work is a core feature of professional autonomy.[13] When medical educators create and implement curricular practices, they also protect how their profession defines and responds to problems, like the equity and empathy problems elaborated above.

Kirch conceptualizes the humanities and social sciences as funda-mental to clinical practice but also as distinctly different from it. The "touchy-feely stuff" entailed in understanding people is contrasted with "scientific knowledge." Thus, in articulating curricular solutions, the medical profession can also articulate their vision of knowledge and what these fields are good for. Curricular practices are ideological.

Second, curricular solutions are appealing in their inordinate promise. Like a professor at the start of summer before preparing a new course for the fall, the details do not need to be ironed out—there is infinite potential for all the brilliant and life-changing les-sons that the professor will impart. At this dreaming phase with the social sciences and humanities in UME, clinical faculty members did not need to define these fields explicitly. They did not need to articu-late a cohesive vision for comprehensive change; the vague curricular solutions seemed enough as simply promises. In fact, the notion that knowledge can solve social problems is a tenet of white liberalism—and reform that is vaguely construed is consistent with the narrative of teleological progress attached to this value.[14] For example, Bernansky, a white male clinical faculty member, gave a vague invocation of the way that the humanities can solve the empathy problems. He told me that, at his school, they were "trying to develop an evidence-based way for the way that humanities, caring, and compassion actually help us advance and improve patient outcomes, lower costs, reduce burn-out, that kind of thing."

Similarly, Dr. Callaghan, a white female clinical faculty member, explained that the reasons for including the humanities were the "increased satisfaction, decreased burnout, increased team cohesion—for the administrators, they care about that. That might mean less turnover. Each time you have to interview and hire a new nurse, new physician, we're talking tens of thousands of dollars. Less sick days." Given how clinical faculty members understand empathy problems, they reduce physician burnout to an individualistic causal chain where the singular physician is burned out, then the physician makes a mistake or is rude to a patient, then the patient is dissatisfied. In this view, the humanities will lead to less burnout, which will lead to patient satisfaction, which in turn will lead to higher reimbursement. It remains unclear, however, *how* the humanities will help.

Again, part of the appeal of the humanities and social sciences is that they can be vaguely promising. Everything is on the table at this curricular dreaming phase—and, as I will show, many schools can remain in this phase with the humanities because the humanities are not required by the governing professional bodies. Many of the medical educators espoused their appreciation for including the humanities and social sciences into their curricular practices and cited wide-ranging reasons, such as:

- Their democratizing implication
- The need to situate the medical profession within broader social-political relationships
- The need for strategies of describing, word choices, arguments for history taking, techniques to ground theories in visual clues, tools to examine how they get to draw to characters and think about stereotypes
- The need to understand what we think we know may change because it is historically and socially situated
- Looking at evidence of disparities based on gender, race, and socioeconomic status

These curricular dreams—what the humanities and social sciences could achieve—are robust. At this stage, the range of potential curricular solutions elaborated in this list also reflects what many of the social scientists and humanists discussed as the merits of integrating their fields into UME curricular practices.

Consequently, at the curricular dreaming phase, I identified three main approaches to conceptualizing the contributions of the social sciences: positivistic (e.g., statistical portrait of social inequalities devoid of context), paternalistic (e.g., imperialistic description of a patient's background), and critical (e.g., contextualized critique of the structural and complex bases of inequalities). The humanities were understood in three central ways: triumphalist (e.g., celebratory understandings of what it means to be a white human), therapeutic (e.g., feel-good tools for coping with dehumanizing conditions), and critical (e.g., historical and reflective critique of the ideas and power structures affecting present-day health and health care). Clinical faculty members were the least likely to espouse critical social science and humanities curricular practices; humanities and social sciences faculty members were the most likely to articulate these approaches.

For example, Dr. Vasquez, a Latino social scientist, worked in a medical school and was trying to develop a critical perspective in medical students. He wanted them to situate their prospective patients in a much bigger social world so that they could better contextualize their patients' health and health care. Vasquez hoped students would approach the clinical encounter with the following set of questions: "Is it something at a cellular or organism level, is it something that's happening within the social behavioral scene, is it within a larger cultural sphere of the institutions within which the patient is embedded or structural types of inequality or disempowerment that are affecting health, or is it the larger fact related to social policy or global environmental factors?" Other social scientists argued for a set of critical curricular practices akin to this.

From the perspective of humanists, the humanities invariably entailed a variety of practices, such as critique, originality, description, appreciation, imagination, provocation, and speculation, to enumerate a few.[15] Within the field of literature alone, stories contain metarepresentation, reconfiguration, perspective taking, and recursive and expansive thought, which Dr. Camara, a Latina humanist, said helped students "appreciate learning how to read critically, learning how to ask critical questions, learning how to listen."[16] Dr. Rogers, a white male humanist, echoed these sentiments and offered an example about the necessity of the humanities for holistically appreciating a patient. He explained that "with an LGBTQ+ patient, a historian would know how this patient population has been treated in the past, their wariness of the medical profession, and even the enduring/ current health problems they incur." Akin to the social scientists, the humanists that were involved with UME curricular practices were advocating for a critical approach to thinking and understanding their patients' social worlds. They centered the patient.

At the dreaming phase, the critical approaches of the humanists and social scientists were amplified when MD-PhDs were given a platform. With the social sciences, Dr. Teatom, a white male MD-PhD with a social sciences degree, explained that the AAMC "had a pretty elementary, shall we say, command of what the social and behavioral sciences were or could be" early in the process of integrating the social sciences into the profession-wide requirements. He was excited by the direction that the profession seemed to be taking, noting, "But we are making progress—I'm on one of the question-writing committees for the National Medical Board Step One and Step Two." By being part of the agenda-setting process of knowledge application, Teatom was poised to actualize critical social science curricular dreams. And in a program report published by the AAMC promoting the "fundamental role" that the humanities played in the instruction of future physicians, the AAMC highlighted the words of Dr. Jeremy Greene, who holds an MD and PhD in history, and is joint appointed at Johns Hopkins: "[H]istorical analysis offers a critical perspective on how medical knowledge is generated, circulated, put to use, and what might be missing from our present structures of medical evidence . . . that historical perspective is crucial to understanding disease, therapeutics, and new technologies as they continually change."[17]

While it makes sense that MD-PhDs with expertise in critical humanistic or social scientific knowledge would dream of curricular practices in a much more expansive way, most clinical faculty members—those who hold most of the curricular power—were by and large not operating in this critical, structural, or reflective mode. Clinical faculty members were more invested in positivistic and paternalistic appreciations of the social sciences, on the one hand, and triumphalist and therapeutic valuations of the humanities, on the other. This is because the valuation of these fields is filtered through clinical faculty members' clinical experience rather than their expertise in these fields.

FROM CURRICULAR DREAMS TO CURRICULAR PROGRAMMING

The medical profession has not stopped short of merely articulating the promises of curricular reform. They have funded research, assembled committees, and suggested curricular programming and requirements that, to differing degrees, incentivize medical schools to include the humanities and social sciences in their curricular practices. For the social sciences, the clinical experiences of clinical faculty members motivated much of their desire to include material. Recall Dr. Pultz, who was introduced earlier in this chapter; she described her clinical faculty chair who realized through clinical practice the extent of the equity problem. Pultz explained that "having come to that realization he spends a lot of time educating around the social determinants of health." Through his "realization" in the clinic, he began to push for including more social sciences, which led to him calling on her expertise. She felt that she was "responding to these needs that people are finding cannot be addressed through basic science or technology or medication alone." As I continued talking with Dr. Li, the clinical faculty member who had a similar realization process as Pultz's chair, Li said that he deliberately sought a residency program in family medicine because it was housed within a department of social medicine. In explaining this choice, he got more excited, stating, "[T]he social medicine, all the population health, advocacy, and all that stuff. I thought, 'Wow this sounds really different, like they're talking about stuff that doesn't even exist in my school.'"[18]

One of the more notable outcomes of the AAMC's curricular committee work on including social scientific material was the addition of sociology to the MCAT in 2015.[19] The group also made recommendations to the Liaison Committee on Medical Education (LCME), the accrediting body of the profession, regarding the instruction of the social sciences in UME training. The LCME standards mandate what medical educators must teach students in UME; otherwise, the medical school risks losing its accreditation. With a rotating twenty-one-member leadership board comprised of seventeen medical educators or practicing physicians, two members of the public, and two medical students operating on a three-year term, the LCME's composition is largely determined by nominations from the AAMC and the American Medical Association (AMA). Every eight years, a school must undergo the accreditation process whereby the school submits an institutional self-study report and then is visited by the LCME survey visit subcommittee to review the assessment of that report.

The LCME standards contain material from several social scientific fields, oriented around the manifestations and underpinnings of social inequalities. There are nine areas in the curricular content section, effective July 1, 2015. I detail four of these areas below:

7.1 BIOMEDICAL, BEHAVIORAL, SOCIAL SCIENCES

The faculty of a medical school ensure that the medical curriculum includes content from the biomedical, behavioral, and socioeconomic sciences to support medical students' mastery of contemporary scientific knowledge and concepts and the methods fundamental to applying them to the health of individuals and populations.

7.2 ORGAN SYSTEMS/LIFE CYCLE/PRIMARY CARE/ PREVENTION/WELLNESS/SYMPTOMS/SIGNS/ DIFFERENTIAL DIAGNOSIS, TREATMENT PLANNING, IMPACT OF BEHAVIORAL/SOCIAL FACTORS

The faculty of a medical school ensure that the medical curriculum includes content and clinical experiences related to each organ system; each phase of the human life cycle; continuity of care; and preventative, acute, chronic, rehabilitative, end-of-life, and primary care in order to prepare students to:

- Recognize wellness, determinants of health, and opportunities for health promotion and disease prevention.
- Recognize and interpret symptoms and signs of disease.
- Develop differential diagnoses and treatment plans.
- Recognize the potential health-related impact on patients of behavioral and socioeconomic factors.
- Assist patients in addressing health-related issues involving all organ systems.

7.5 SOCIETAL PROBLEMS

The faculty of a medical school ensure that the medical curriculum includes instruction in the diagnosis, prevention, appropriate reporting, and treatment of the medical consequences of common societal problems.

7.6 CULTURAL COMPETENCE/HEALTH CARE DISPARITIES/PERSONAL BIAS

The faculty of a medical school ensure that the medical curriculum provides opportunities for medical students to learn to recognize and appropriately address gender and cultural biases in themselves, in others, and in the health care delivery process. The medical curriculum includes instruction regarding:

- The manner in which people of diverse cultures and belief systems perceive health and illness and respond to various symptoms, diseases and treatments.
- The basic principles of culturally competent health care.
- The recognition and development of solutions for health care disparities.
- The importance of meeting the health care needs of medically underserved populations.
- The development of core professional attributes (e.g., altruism, accountability) needed to provide effective care in a multidimensionally diverse society.

These LCME standards simultaneously conflate different social sciences disciplines—for example, the "socioeconomic sciences" in section 7.1—and draw on positivistic and paternalistic approaches to social science. Section 7.2, with its vague emphasis on "social factors," section 7.5 and the general language of "the medical consequences of common societal problems," and section 7.6, with its similarly unelaborated requirement for "personal bias" and "cultural competence" all contribute to a lack of attention to context and systems while illuminating individual-level dynamics and highlighting the otherness of patients that are from "diverse cultures and belief systems."[20] That said, the LCME are requiring some content and are an opening, an opportunity.

The AAMC has engaged in a few profession-wide initiatives with the humanities. While not required, there are professional investments and energy behind their incorporation. For example, the AAMC funded a new initiative, the Fundamental Role of Arts and Humanities in Medical Education (FRAHME). FRAHME was designed to "provide resources to help medical educators start, develop, and/or improve the use of the arts and humanities in their teaching."

This FRAHME initiative ran on the heels of the Project to Rebalance and Integrate Medical Education (PRIME), wherein medical educators aimed to utilize the humanities within UME to promote empathy, virtue, genuineness, and self-awareness.[21] In addition to establishing grant funding for these curricular programs, the AAMC published a monograph about the need and commitment to these programs, a guidebook with exemplary programs, and a professional development program oriented around the evaluation and assessment of these programs. In introducing this initiative, AAMC president and CEO Dr. Darrell G. Kirch claimed that "at the AAMC, we are looking to build a case to medical educators that this is integral to what we do." Here, Kirch framed the humanities as foundational to clinical practice.

Thus, at the discursive level, the profession-wide curricular dreams show a robust potential for the humanities in medical education. In an AAMC press release on the state of the humanities in medical education, the AAMC's position was that "arts and humanities are essential to the human experience and their benefits to medical education go far beyond joys and pleasures. By integrating arts and humanities throughout medical education, trainees and physicians can learn to be better observers and interpreters; and build empathy, communication and teamwork skills, and more." As the AAMC chief medical education officer Dr. Alison Whelan has stated, however, there has not been a "deep, sustained, foundational, across-the-board incorporation into all medical schools."[22] Not only has there been a lack of across-the-board incorporation, but the way that the clinical faculty appreciate the need for the humanities has already started to limit their potential contributions.

Dr. Schumann, introduced earlier in this chapter, described the contribution of the humanities to medicine as being about "how we are human and how we might care for each other and ourselves." She offered her construction of the solution, saying that the "humanities offers ways to reflect and to think—it can actually help alleviate the suffering of our medical students and physicians—the humanities gives them tools to be able to deal with the suffering that they see, to deal with the monstrous things that they are asked to do to human bodies." The humanities here were conflated with "what it is like to be human" without regard for how humanists themselves constructed the value of their fields. Dr. George, also introduced earlier in this chapter, had tapped into the way the humanities were conceptualized as necessary for giving students the ability to create the conditions under which "it feels like" they had meaning in their work.

In sum, the first step for the medical profession's curricular dreams to become curricular realities is for the creation of curricular requirements and programming. Medical educators at the national, professional level have vocalized—and, in some cases, incentivized—the desire for physicians to cultivate better communication skills; understand the patient as a whole person; be sensitive to a wide range of beliefs about health, illness, and treatment; and identify and address rampant health and health-care inequities.[23] The primacy of clinical experience already began to constrain the curricular dreams (internally) at this phase because there were alternate framings of problems and solutions from students and other faculty members (externally) that could be more critical and structural. But even with curricular dreams, the clinical faculty members' voices were the loudest.

PROFESSION-WIDE PRESSURES TO ADOPT NEW CURRICULAR PRACTICES

The twin crises around inhumane and inequitable care were certainly at the forefront of my respondents' minds and the profession-wide reports; they felt that these were serious equity and empathy problems in need of curricular solutions. A cynical interpretation of these curricular dreams would be that these clinical faculty members were simply engaged in public relations—a take that sociologists have argued before.[24] I believe that many, if not most, clinical faculty members were sincerely responding to their perception of equity and empathy problems; however, a few medical educators in my study were interested in incorporating the humanities and social sciences because they wanted to be competitive in the broader medical education field.

This competitive spirit was apparent at the annual AAMC meetings, where medical schools—and individual educators—vied for prestige. Most telling was the question-and-answer period after panel presentations, which often took on a "this is more of a comment than a question" character. A medical educator, usually a clinical faculty member, would raise their hand or approach the microphone and begin by introducing themselves, their position, their experience, and their school. "I am So and So from XYZ and have [number of] years in this role and [number of] years in that role." They would then proceed to tell the audience what they do for their curricular practices at their school. The degree to which their example fit the panel at hand varied. In this sense, these clinical faculty members seemed less interested in learning about curricular practices and more invested in performing what their school was up to—this was particularly the case for the humanities sessions.

In interviews, many clinical faculty members described their humanities and social sciences offerings with immense pride. They described their program as "by far the largest, most prestigious, most extensive, most long-standing." They noted how "totally off the charts in terms of U.S. medical schools" their humanities curricular practices were. They claimed that their "extensive" social sciences curriculum was "one of the reasons students came" to their school. The notion that curricular strength in the social sciences and humanities was a "selling point" for medical schools was common, even if their school did not have the kind of curricular practices they wanted. In fact, when I asked Dr. Brown, a white male humanist, whether there were any faculty members he had to convince of the importance of his humanities curriculum, he explained that "the head of admissions has told me on numerous occasions 'you know this is a great recruiting tool—I mean all of the prospective medical students love it, they find it so interesting that you're doing this at the medical school, they never see this at any of the other medical schools.'" Brown concluded his answer by telling me, "[I]t's like a recruiting tool for our institutions, so you know it's just the opposite of having to convince people."

Where Brown had been told by his school's head of admissions that their curricular practices set them apart from other schools, schools where faculty members might want to get curricular practices off the ground might also make curricular decisions with one eye on the broader field and another on their available resources. Dr. Stern, a white female clinical faculty member at another medical school, elaborated on how the broader field affected her ability to incorporate new humanities material, saying that when their school saw that "something like this is popular—we did a little bit of research and found that a number of medical schools have programs like that—that was influential." She went on to say how they "had to show that we had people willing to donate, you know, all the things that the school looked for—does it come with prestige or money?" At Stern's school, the status of the humanities curricular material was pivotal to its acceptance by the leadership.

Students picked up on how some of these curricular practices seemed to be in vogue. One Latina student, Nina, told me why she thought her medical school offered a humanities elective by saying, "I think that it is very important in medical school dialogue, like the dialogue around changing curriculum, *to say* that you are having humanities foci now." After saying this, her eyes widened, and she continued, with a hint of sarcasm, "[E]ven research schools are saying we want our doctors to be humans first because they feel this kind of pressure to make sure that the students they are training become not only good doctors but good people, too." To Nina's point, larger groups are oriented around promoting the incorporation of the humanities into medical school curricular practices. The website of a profession-wide group called the Health Humanities Consortium (HHC) has a page dedicated to a "marketing strategy template." In the pitch for the pitch, the HHC claims that the strategy is aimed at showing "why students will choose your program over the competitor institutions." Both my respondents and the HHC are speaking about schools who are trying to be competitive in the medical education field.

The profession itself stokes this vision of this humanities curricular programming as a mark of distinction and as a recruiting tool to attract specific future doctors in ways that are reminiscent of the humanities as pedigree discourse during the mid-twentieth century. But it is a mixed group of schools that advertise with these numbers: for example, when the *U.S. News & Reports* issued a news release highlighting schools that had 19 to 33 percent of the incoming cohort of medical students majoring in humanities or social sciences, not all the schools had Ivy League prestige.[25] Taking the marketing angle one step further and speaking to the degree to which clinical faculty members drive these curricular practices, some physicians developed notoriety for their work and led faculty development trainings and workshops for faculty members from other schools to come learn from the "experts" on these curricular practices. Not only did this entrepreneurial spirit enable the clinical faculty members to have control over these curricular practices, but it also solidified the association between the branded curricular practices and a famous faculty member's school on the national stage. Medical school leadership looking out for their material and symbolic interests could be understood as showing interest convergence, where the dominant group only makes a change if their interests align with it, or health equity tourism, where previously uncommitted researchers tap into new funding streams to boost their careers or their school's profile.[26]

* * *

Whether medical educators were incorporating the humanities and social sciences out of a genuine desire to improve curricular practices—and ultimately clinical practices—or out of a wish to sig-nal status, they were participating in a profession-wide discussion about what these curricular practices could and should look like. Emerging from these curricular dreaming discussions was a profile of a physician who must know the social context of their patients and hone their interpretive and observational knowledge and skills for the clinic. Sure enough, there is evidence that engagement with the humanities and social sciences can allow physicians to provide more empathic and equitable attitudes.[27] Even though these profession-wide needs, dreams, and programming for these curricular practices were coalescing around a set of ideas about what a good physician looked like, the process by which these bodies of knowledge could be applied still remained rather nebulous, and these curricular dreams were still quite vague. This vague character was important to the appeal of these fields for curricular reform. They could be anything the clinical faculty members wanted them to be. But in addition, the other side of the flexible curricular dreaming coin rendered the prag-matic enactment of curricular reform rather unclear.

3

DESIGNING CURRICULAR PRACTICES AT EACH MEDICAL SCHOOL

F inding the medical educators in charge of curricular practices was often a convoluted journey. After scouring websites
to find these educators, I then had to locate them physically,
traversing through the bowels of buildings. That is how I found
Dr. Kling, a white male course director of the undergraduate medical education (UME) curriculum. He was a physician by training
and had come into this position of leadership after years of clinical experience, saying of his role, "I sorta just fell into it." Because
he was a course director, I asked him whether any social sciences or
humanities were taught at his school. In response, Kling pulled up
the Liaison Committee on Medical Education (LCME) standards
and began reading them off verbatim to me. After he quoted the
LCME Standard 7.1, described in the previous chapter, he said:

> When they send out self-study documents, curricula come under these
> categories: biomedical informatics, complementary alternative health
> care, evidence-based medicine, global health issues, health-care financ-
> ing, human development/life cycle, human sexuality, law in medicine,
> medication management/compliance, medical socioeconomics, nutri-
> tion, pain management, palliative care, patient safety, and population-
> based medicine. And they ask: "Is it taught as an independent course or
> an integrated course, and in which years is it taught?"

Kling then went on to read LCME Standard 7.5, also described in chapter 2, and explained how that standard was "still being increasingly defined as to whether you talk about issues of food deserts and poverty and gangs, or different social and environmental determinants of health. And so that's an area in evolution."

As we continued our discussion, Kling continued to recite these LCME standards, verbatim. He concluded with the rhetorical remark, "[A] lot of stuff, right?" He was proud of what was contained in these professional guidelines, thinking that this was a step in the right direction. The majority of the medical educators—clinical faculty members and humanities and social sciences faculty members— I interviewed for this project perceived the LCME standards to be a positive development. At first glance, these standards, with their requirements and follow-up assessment, seem promising. They do look like "a lot of stuff." Indeed, research on organizational reform suggests that reforms are often doomed to fail without the teeth that incentivize the reformative action, so the mere presence of these professional guidelines is an important measure for incorporating the social sciences.[1] Scholars of organizational reform, however, also point to the importance of clarity and specificity in standards—the more vague a requirement, the more open to interpretation a requirement, the more likely a change in requirement will fail to enact the change it was meant to address.[2]

The LCME standards represent the good intentions of the medical profession; they also embody the kernels of curricular failures. My interview with Kling is emblematic here. He was beaming over the promise of these LCME standards; he found these professional guidelines to be important and something that he and his colleagues took seriously. They wanted to address the equity problems facing their profession and enact the LCME standards. But his remarks also highlight the organizational and epistemic seeds of failure. By saying "a lot of stuff," Kling showed the gargantuan task ahead for curricular designers at each medical school. They needed to make decisions about what to teach, how to teach it, and when to teach it. With his comments about topical areas that were being "increasingly defined" or an "area in evolution," Kling pointed to how the LCME standards were very much open to interpretation. The ambiguity seed of failure also begets another seed of failure: that of *who* was doing the defining and interpreting of these ambiguous standards. While I cannot know for certain why he quoted the LCME standards verbatim to me, the fact that Kling needed to read them aloud—rather than paraphrase or explain them—denotes a lack of expertise with the topical material. In his "a lot of stuff" list, structural inequalities like racism and heteronormativity were notably absent.

Thus, just as there was palpable enthusiasm for these curricular practices in the abstract, there was also a pronounced uncertainty among medical educators, especially clinical faculty members, about how to proceed. They did not know, exactly, how to implement them. I witnessed this collective confusion and organizational decoupling at one session at the 2016 annual meeting of the Association of American Medical Colleges (AAMC). A panelist discussing how to approach the instruction of social sciences in UME presented on the LCME standards. They closed their presentation by saying, "LCME accreditation data is not publicly available because it is probably *so bad*." The audience burst out in knowing laughter. The panelist went on to give suggestions on how to improve the inclusion of the social sciences in UME for the interested audiences, but the general acceptance of this failure was telling.

At another AAMC annual meeting in 2017, I observed a panel on incorporating the humanities into the curriculum. A presenter described how, in an ideal scenario, they would teach a course on the history of medicine for all medical students; they would focus on the importance of understanding the past to help envision the physician's role in the present. The clinical faculty members who were presenting then offered practical implementation suggestions for the attendees in the audience that would be feasible with their budgets and personnel, suggestions that vastly reduced the time and engagement with the discipline of history. For example, they suggested that schools could create celebrations for big historical events or have students talk to older faculty members about their experiences training. The clinical faculty members in this audience all nodded their heads in agreement, as if these examples of inclusions of "history" would be the same thing as learning the critical lessons that historians have about the knowledge production and practices of the medical profession.[3] The distinction I am trying to make is that learning about how a white male emeritus faculty member understood his career is very different then learning about how J. Marion Sims tortured and exploited Black women in developing gynecological procedures.

In panel after panel, as well as in my interviews with medical educators, the task of taking the promise of these curricular dreams and transforming them into tangible curricular practices was fraught with a host of challenges. The social sciences and humanities have slightly different processes of knowledge application, considering that the former was required and the latter was not; given how the LCME standards are still very much "standards in evolution," however, both fields were subject to the same interpretive work done by the same people: clinical faculty members. In this chapter, I review the organizational and epistemic barriers that curricular designers confronted when they attempted to take professional guidelines and design curricular practices at their home institution. I show how the disorganization of the medical school created the conditions under which there was very little oversight over the curriculum and white clinical faculty members had outsized influence on shaping these practices. When medical educators mapped out what, how, and when to teach the social sciences and humanities, they made consequential decisions about what constituted knowledge, who was worthy of being admitted into medical school, and how to reinforce the status quo of the profession, whether they realized it or not.

THE DISORGANIZATION AND FACULTY COMPOSITION OF THE U.S. MEDICAL SCHOOL

Many of the foundational studies within the sociology of medical education depict the medical profession as one homogenous unit. In some instances, this assumption of homogeneity is methodological because scholars abstracted from a case study of a single school, thus missing the heterogeneity.[4] But the assumption of homogeneity is also pivotal to the theoretical conceptualization of professions. Whether through the standardization of the educational requirements or the acquisition of expert knowledge around a specific set of tasks and problems, unified standards were—and are—key to the medical profession's claim to legitimacy.[5] Despite the existence of variation, therefore, the promise of homogeneity is part and parcel of the status of medicine as a profession.

But this homogeneity was far afield from the perceived curricular reality of those charged with designing and implementing curricular practices. Medical educators loved to joke, as one panelist at an AAMC annual meeting remarked, that "if you've seen one medical school you've seen one medical school." There was a pervasive sentiment among my respondents that each school was different from the others, or, as a white male social scientist who worked at a medical school, Dr. Warner, remarked, "[E]very school is going to have to find their own model and what works with their local culture and their faculty." Perhaps most exemplative here was what I learned at a session on the humanities in medical education at an AAMC annual meeting in 2015. Before the session started, I asked a medical educator at my table whether she organized any humanities curriculum at her home institution. Her reply stuck with me, especially given how it reverberated across the conference and in interviews. She said, "[O]h, medical schools don't *organize* . . . they respond to crises . . . we do crisis management." And Dr. Bettles, a white female social scientist at one medical school, echoed this participant's remarks about the crisis mentality, saying that "in medicine I think one of the big things is that there is a lot of like dike-plugging with the finger as opposed to like zooming out and saying like, '[W]hat's going on.' That's my biggest frustration with my field and my department."

What I think these respondents are addressing is that curricular practices are a flexible template for each medical school to absorb crises and maintain their status quo, whether that status quo is in the social composition of the profession or the epistemic perspective of the physician. To help explain this claim, I first must show the *organizational flexibility* built into leaders' approaches to organizing and hiring medical educators tasked with mapping the curricular practices at medical schools. By "organizational flexibility," I mean that medical schools, as organizations, are structured with the freedom of choice and with unspecified processes contained within their operations. Organizations that sustain professions encourage flexibility to cultivate the autonomous professional but also because flexibility is a feature of the twenty-first-century organization governed by bureaucratic and capitalistic priorities.[6]

The physical layout of medical schools both structures and symbolizes the organizational flexibility—or, as some of my respondents described it, chaos. These places were physically disorienting, with expanding, sprawling, and fragmented compositions of buildings, old and new.[7] In the course of my research, I often went to schools to conduct interviews in person, either with educators or students. I visited dozens of them. So much of my logistical experience in trying to carry out the interviews mirrored how I was trying to make sense of the subject matter. Where is this building? How can I find it? What do you mean this person's office has moved but you now don't know where it is? The offices of my respondents were in all sorts of areas—it was rare that the relevant medical educators' offices were in a centralized location for medical education. Many of the individual offices were nothing to write home about: they often received very little light, were tucked in behind a lab, or were located on a random floor. The exceptions were the offices of the bigwig deans, who often had much more fancy accommodations. I often felt lost and confused in trying to find a particular person.

This disorienting feeling had the effect of making it not totally clear who was in charge, which educator did what, and especially how collaboration worked. It obscured who was in power. Many respondents remarked on how siloed they were and how difficult it was finding the time, space, or right person with whom to collaborate. Medical schools were fractals of the AAMC annual medical education conferences— overwhelming, overlapping, disjointed—which elicited a sense of confusion and intimidation. Only the people in the know seemed comfortable with these arrangements. Most of these offices and the AAMC annual meetings were removed from spaces where patient contact could occur or often where educational activities would happen. Those in charge of designing curricular practices and implementing professional standards were thus both disorganized and obscured from the view of their constituents.

Just as the spatial infrastructure was a compilation of parts with a confusing design that was more of an afterthought, so, too, was the organizational infrastructure of medical schools. Medical schools sported a highly complex organizational structure.[8] Senior leadership, with deans, varied in number and levels. Sometimes a medical school had a dedicated office for medical education; others had just the UME or graduate medical education (GME) senior leadership and course directors. Most medical schools had offices of student affairs; faculty affairs; research; and diversity, equity, and inclusion. In line with administrative expansion across academic settings, medical schools have been increasingly expanding their administrative structure with more and more positions, and the AAMC annual meetings reflect this, with target sections and sessions for particular positions (e.g., deans, course directors) and tasks (e.g., curricular design, assessment, faculty development).[9] Clinical faculty members comprise the bulk of these positions, including those overseeing the curricular design and everyday instruction of medical students.

Clinical faculty members are by far the largest group employed full-time by medical schools, at roughly 89 percent.[10] As this group maintains professional dominance so, too, do white people. Recent reports from the AAMC faculty roster documented how much the number of clinical faculty grew, more than doubling in size from 1990 to 2016; in that same time period, Black and Latinx clinical faculty underrepresentation *increased* across sixteen clinical specialties at all professor levels (e.g., assistant, associate, full), with the exception of Black women in obstetrics and gynecology.[11] While roughly just 10 percent of the medical school faculties are basic sciences faculty at medical schools, they have been and remain majority white and male, and this is particularly the case for associate and full professors.[12] The remaining 1 percent of medical school faculties in the United States are comprised of scholars from "other" disciplines, like the humanities, social sciences, or education.

While there were no systematic data about the 1 percent of "other" scholars, many of my respondents from humanities and social sciences backgrounds noted that they also fell into these positions by happenstance, just like Dr. Kling, the clinical faculty member introduced at the beginning of the chapter, articulated. White male humanist Dr. Rogers explained, "I think a lot of people who 'just' have a PhD in a humanities or social sciences field who are appointed as professors in the medical school are surprised they are there or think that this was not a part of their original plan." Or as another respondent, Dr. Pultz, a white female social scientist, stated, "[I]f you would have told me that I would be a professor in a medical school, I would have been like, '[Y]ou are shitting me.' I was resoundingly antagonistic, like, 'fuck you, medicine' as a graduate student studying the field." It makes sense that these humanities and social sciences faculty members were simply falling into these positions given that there was no organized professional movement to try and populate medical schools with scholars from these fields.

From the available pool of (mostly) clinical faculty members, a certain coterie of them at each medical school become involved in making decisions about curricular content at the UME level and also at the individual course level. Recall how my tablemate at the AAMC conference said, "[W]e don't organize, we respond to crises." While there are some positions that are advertised and formal hiring processes ensue, so many of my respondents spoke of an informal, disorganized way that they fell into their role, just like Dr. Kling, Dr. Rogers, and Dr. Pultz. I want to take a moment here and say that many clinical faculty members who fell into these roles seemed to do so out of a sense of duty. There was an immediate organizational need and they filled it, often at personal cost (e.g., time, money, sanity). But the informality and haphazard approach to filling UME (and other medical education) positions at medical schools meant that white clinical faculty members were more likely to be hired and that there was no overarching plan for them when they assumed their role.[13]

Therefore, many positions at medical schools came with greater oversight, like attendings and program directors, and others less so, like those facilitating small-group sessions. Some of the clinical faculty members who took on these paid roles in curricular design did them in limited capacities, like a three-year appointment at 25 percent time. Most of the clinical faculty members did not have training in these organizational, pedagogical, and administrative tasks. In addition, they had other components to their job that took 75 percent of their time, like seeing patients or engaging in research; teaching was the smallest and least compensated part of their work. Many clinical faculty members that I spoke to who had a part-time appointment routinely worked more hours in the week than they were paid for. In addition, there were many other positions where clinical faculty members taught as volunteers, viewing this labor as both an obligation to the profession and an honor to be selected. This volunteer corps tended to lead the small-group sessions and electives.

The final component to the disorganization of U.S. medical schools was the degree of personnel turnover. There was a revolving door of part-time and volunteer clinical faculty members working as medical educators. Thus, clinical faculty members often cycled through these positions of curricular power with no explicit expertise and no time to develop (let alone enforce) a unifying vision for the courses. In these cases, there was very little overarching curricular development and faculty expertise, pointing to a seemingly chaotic organizational infrastructure. It was no wonder that my respondents spoke so often of crises. To illustrate further how the disorganization of medical schools placed clinical faculty members in curricular power, take the experiences of some of the medical educators I interviewed for my project. They spoke about how the payment structure, scheduling differences, and research priorities placed humanities and social sciences faculty members in marginalized positions relative to the clinical faculty, the only exception being if the clinical faculty *also* had a degree in a social sciences or humanities discipline.

Dr. Wright, a white male MD-PhD, elaborated on the organizational structure of his medical school. He said that the payment structure of the clinical versus academic track could allow him to do "half-time clinical work and then basically *volunteer work* as an academic because the half-time clinical salaries are essentially the equivalent to full-time academic salaries of junior faculty." He continued, "[Y]ou had complete job security because there's no physician unemployment in the United States. As long as you have any credibility as a scholar you know programs will be happy to have a competent person *teaching for free*." Clinical faculty members were the most flexible given how the bulk of their salaries were paid through their clinical revenue stream. In referring to the "volunteer" research he did, Wright underscored the dominant assumption that clinical salaries are sufficient, further reinforcing that clinical faculty members are the ones in charge and the leaders at medical schools were interested in having faculty teach "for free."

Faculty members like Wright were quite helpful for their school's curricular practices because of their reimbursement flexibility. Not every school had this reserve of dual-degreed faculty to draw from. When I asked about challenges to the inclusion of humanities or social sciences at their school, white male clinical faculty member Dr. Engle explained to me, "[T]he obstacle ends up being not interest or understanding of the importance of the opportunity, but more just kind of funding logistics. It turns out that the incentive systems for the medical school and the undergraduate institution are really misaligned, and it's actually difficult for the undergraduate system to pay me in the coin of my realm, or for the medical school to pay an anthropologist in the coin of their realm." Unless they also had a clinical credential, faculty members with expertise in other fields were less exploitable within the medical school because of how academic appointments operated. Some professors—particularly those from social sciences or humanities backgrounds—did not want to take on curricular design tasks because, quite simply, the committee work was not reimbursed or rewarded by their department. As a social scientist on the tenure track in a department of medical education, Dr. Bettles needed to protect herself and did not go as far as she wanted to with curricular matters. She explained:

> I think there needs to be lot more and I'm protecting myself as an untenured person and not teaching an elective. Whereas I could and they would want me to, but I'm not doing that because that's not expected of me, so I'm not doing it. So I don't pipe up from the audience very often and correct people or things like that, which is something I would want to do maybe but I can't. But my job is mainly research and because I'm focused on research, it's not as much on the curriculum.

In concluding her remarks, Bettles mentioned that "in general the med school stuff I've learned on the job and I think it is really important to be good at doing ethnography of real life for this." Like Bettles,

Dr. Grossmith, a white female social scientist at a different medical school, had become attuned to the incentive structures in place. She pointed out that curricular work was often not something that she could justify pursuing given her junior faculty status and career interests and, to harken back to what Engle said, given the funding logistics in the "coin of [her] realm." Although Grossmith wanted to teach a course on the critical social sciences, she said that she "intentionally" did not take over "developing and implementing the curriculum on social topics in the med school because [she's] on a different calendar and the calendar's really different." For Grossmith, the structure of appointments and attendant calendars (e.g., the academic year for the medical school starts July 1; it starts around September 1 for the social sciences department) did not give her the time or the incentive to participate in curricular development despite possessing the expertise.

Research priorities also reinforced the clinical faculty members' power. Dr. Vasquez, a Latino social scientist, elaborated that, at his school, "there's this powerful medical education unit here that is really junk. You look at the research, it's just totally junk and if you've been trained, good methodological training as a sociologist, I'm like this is crap." He went on to say how those clinical faculty members "passed judgment on our curriculum using the stupidest metric imaginable. They just come up with this stuff and then measure it bizarrely, and then they do these sloppy before-and-after comparisons and you're just like, what the—without any sense of what is our measurement model and what are we really trying to get at. It's populated mostly by people who have an MD." The sense that clinical faculty members were dominant—and that their judgment was suspect—pervaded the experiences that humanities and social sciences faculty members shared with me.

These humanities and social sciences scholars were adept at recognizing the dominance of the clinical faculty in these spaces and tried to navigate within those constraints. One white female social scientist, Dr. Geronimos, described how during their postdoctoral work, they became fascinated watching "how curriculum was being conceptualized, like the debates around what constitutes relevance, what do we mean, like who gets the resources if we think of teaching as symbolic capital. Those fights between the different constituents— and they were very collegial—but they reminded me a lot of political state-type of relationships." Thus, some humanities and social sciences educators described the skill it took in "sneaking in" more critical work from their home disciplines, like teaching about how biomedicine itself is a culture or how the emotional socialization of medical students is steeped in dehumanizing rhetoric. Dr. Payne, a white female social scientist, looked at sneaking in social science in a much more strategic way, by convincing the field of medical education that they had come up with the idea in the first place.

As Payne recounted, "[M]edicine is so widely powerful that these types of subtleties of what's political science or sociology, they don't even have to think about that stuff. They're just like, whatever, we see something, we take it. They're so progressively dominant and so I feel like the key is to try to trick them into thinking that this thing that came out of sociology is actually something that a MD said." In explaining to me how they act strategically in faculty or decision-making meetings, white male social scientist Dr. Warner said how "now, I'm like, 'okay, if I can get what I want using your words, because I know it's the same thing, and I can sort of more covertly throw it in there, I'm happy.'" Payne and Warner thus recalled a strategy or social skill that educators like them used—they both played to clinical relevance and the dominance of the medical profession itself.

FROM ORGANIZATIONAL CHAOS
TO CURRICULAR DESIGN

Medical school leaders, with their decisions about reimbursement and faculty composition, created the conditions in which there was very little organization and a dominance of white clinical faculty members in positions of curricular power. The clinical faculty members in charge of curricular design had to interpret, organize, and distribute curricular practices at their individual medical school. In both cases, the clinical faculty had standards or programming to refer to in their decision making, where they were trying to figure out where and when to include social sciences and humanities content.

Designing and implementing curricular reform is not easy, despite the outcomes of decisions being important. Dr. Rivas, a Latino clinician and social scientist (MD-PhD), had been trying to create a longitudinal course on critical race theory at his medical school. He specifically wanted students to interrogate the race-based medicine they were otherwise uncritically consuming, like the race-based adjustment with kidney function levels. When I asked what seemed to be in his way, he chuckled, saying: "[T]here's all kinds of barriers to any piece of anything you want to include. There's time, there's money, there's buy-in; three pretty good ones. Time, money, buy-in. People don't want to do it, or don't have the time to do it, or there are not the resources to support doing it. Other than that, it's an almost flawless plan." His sarcastic closing to what he was up against seemed par for the course in the context of most U.S. medical schools, where there were several epistemic and organizational barriers to including the humanities and social sciences as critical curricular practices.

The barriers stemmed sometimes from the disorganization itself. As Dr. Brown, a white male humanist, noted, "I mean I know what I teach in my course, but I don't know what's taught in the other courses that are also offered. Trying to figure out who knows everything and figuring out a way of tracking that is surprisingly challenging. You have to have a good database that you can search to say, '[A]ll right, cultural competency appears in lecture one in this course and in lecture five in that course and this learning objective is here and there.'" According to white female clinical faculty member Dr. Gartland, the lack of organization makes it so that the faculty members in charge of putting together their school's curricular practices must contend with "fifteen people wanting air-time for a single lesson slot but no vision from those on high."

Regarding the buy-in factor from the barriers that Rivas outlined, outright rejection of social science writ large was rare, in part because of the backing of the professional bodies and the institutional isomorphic pressures for schools to conform.[14] Those who were depicted as needing buy-in were not clinical faculty members but basic sciences faculty members. I will give an extended example from my conversation with Dr. Li, an Asian male clinical faculty member who oversaw his school's UME, who elaborated about how he approached integrating the social sciences into his school's curricular practices. Li had told me that they were initially fighting folks for space in the curriculum to have topics such as "community health, occupational health, environmental health, health policy, health disparities, and social determinants of health." In "heading two of the subcommittees," Li felt that he was "running around with templates and crazy stuff" because he was trying to capitalize on the interest within the profession as well as at his school. Despite the interest from his fellow clinical faculty members in including these topics for the past dozen years, he said, very little had made its way into his school's curricular practices. He was really excited by the LCME standards, telling me, "[A]ctually requiring the teaching of population health, requiring the teaching of implicit bias . . . I mean all of the stuff that I've been saying forever. Thank God they finally put that in there so we have to teach it." Li felt that, with the LCME standards, they finally had the impetus to get that material in, but he also described some significant barriers that he still faced.

Li felt that it was the basic sciences faculty members who perceived their disciplinary knowledge to be under threat and who were blocking meaningful curricular change. He parodied some basic sciences faculty member on his curricular reconfiguration subcommittee, saying "[O]h, my six weeks of molecular biology signify that I'm somehow not as important as a block that is twelve weeks in length."

Li went on to say, "[S]o when you're trying to teach something like population health that was never a part of the curriculum at all and it wasn't seen as important the people who are going to complain the most are—and again these are just general rules but it's the truth—the basic sciences faculty are absolutely the first ones to panic. Because the trend in every medical school is that you're shortening the basic science years." Many of my respondents also spoke of basic sciences faculty the way that Li did, pointing to those faculty members as the first ones to balk at including social sciences and humanities content at their fields' potential expense.

As Li gestures to, faculty members perceived the amount of time allotted to a particular organ or biochemical process as a statement about their importance to the profession. When curricular designers were making decisions about changing the curriculum, they were balancing people's egos as well as the limits of time. Latina clinical faculty member Dr. Gutierrez relayed this impression by stating, "I believe that most faculty see the value of the courses. They just don't want to give up time in their own course for another course." While some basic sciences faculty members might be panicking about their relevance, other basic sciences faculty members might question the relevance of the humanities and social sciences altogether. When incorporating social sciences into an environment where, as South Asian female clinical faculty member Dr. Shah said, "within the world of medicine you need to mitigate countervailing messages that say this is a waste of your time," educators described needing to overcome attitudes of basic sciences faculty members that the humanities and social sciences are useless, soft, or too critical in order for the basic sciences faculty members to give up some of their curricular time.

Given that basic sciences faculty comprise roughly 10 percent of the full-time faculty positions at medical schools, I found it curious that they were constructed as such a fall guy. While it may be "the truth," as Li put it, that they were the stubborn barnacles on the ships of curricular progress, they were also a convenient foe.

They were professionally distinct from the clinical faculty members, obviating the medical profession of blame for curricular failure. They also held very little curricular power, in terms of numbers as well as influence, because the clinical faculty members hold the power. Although the clinical faculty members tended to paint the basic sciences faculty members as the scapegoats for stymying their curricular reform, the real issues stemmed from the way in which the clinical faculty members understood the relevance of social scientific and humanistic knowledge. Their interpretations were crucial for patterning curricular design, at times at the expense of other disciplines or professions.[15] With little to no training in pedagogy, their clinical experiences were their central link to relevance.

While clinical relevance mattered for their approach to both equity and empathy problems, I call the process by which clinical faculty members simultaneously appreciated the reality of social inequalities while fundamentally misunderstanding the social scientific study of them *clinical witnessing*. Dr. Wright, the MD-PhD introduced earlier in this chapter, argued that the key to "hooking" the stubborn basic sciences faculty members was by leveraging clinical relevance:

> For the average clinician what you can learn by studying history is actually pragmatically more useful than a lot of the basic science that you'll learn. When the basic science faculty hear that at first they just dismiss it right out. But if you can engage them in the conversation in the day-to-day life of a primary care clinician whose lessons are really more valuable for them . . . if they're thoughtful, they will eventually yield the case because you just don't need to know that much anatomy.

Dr. Watkins, a white male clinical educator, explained that his impetus for wanting to add social sciences to the curriculum "was experiential—it was the lived experience that forced, I think, me at the time to really look more critically from our perspective as the physician and what we brought to the table with us affected how we cared for patients." Watkins points to his clinical experience as paramount, just as Dr. Krebs, another white male clinical faculty member, did. In articulating why the LCME standards must be taught, Krebs said:

> If you're awake and alert, you realize, 'ufff if I write for something and they can't afford it, then what's the point?' Or if I don't take the moment to hear them when they say they're tired or they're hurt or whatever. You know you have to stop and try to understand what that means to that person, and then that's not fluffy and it's not soft it's—it is what it is because it happens to people.

With the audible acknowledgement of the potential futility of prescribing medication to a patient who cannot afford it, Krebs's "ufff" captures just how important he thought it was for clinicians to bear witness to the social factors affecting their patients. He also denoted how this importance is obvious to anyone paying attention, to anyone "awake and alert."

Similarly, when Dr. Tortora, a white male course director of the practice of medicine (POM) sequence at his medical school, explained the importance of the POM course content on the social sciences to me, he said: "I think anyone who's worked in a health-care setting knows that on an individual day, you're going to see people that you would never see in your day-to-day life. No two people are the same—what motivates them, what drives them, what resources they have. I may see, on a given day, a Syrian refugee with nothing. Literally nothing. And then see a hedge fund manager who has 500 houses." By leading with "anyone who's worked in a health-care setting knows," Tortora was also invoking the ubiquity of clinical experiences with social difference and why the LCME standards on the social sciences were clinically relevant. Tortora pointed to how these clinical experiences were based on what they witness rather than their personal lived experience because most clinical faculty members were from socially privileged backgrounds and the patients were people they would "never see" in their "day-to-day lives."[16]

As I will describe in the next section, this epistemic perspective held by clinical faculty members—and made possible by the (dis) organization of the medical school—was very consequential for the decisions they made in designing the curriculum. Clinical experience is *not* knowledge about the historical origins or contemporary manifestations of social inequalities. Not only were they constructing a heroic narrative around their awareness in relation to the backward basic sciences faculty members, but with this clinical witnessing the clinical faculty members were also patterning the delivery of material.

SHOEHORNING IN THE SOCIAL SCIENCES

Early in the course of my interview with Dr. Perez, a Latino social scientist, I asked him a general question about how his particular medical school approached the incorporation of the social sciences and humanities. Like others, he laughed. He then started by explaining to me that "there hasn't been a coherent overarching idea in terms of integration of either humanities or social science sets of lectures or even sets of activities that all students are required to do." He half-smiled and raised his eyebrows, expressing disappointment as he continued: "[T]here's a *smattering* in doctoring—there is something on, like, the social determinants of health—but there isn't nearly as much there and it's hard to tell exactly where it is because it's sort of slipped in in ways that are often *invisible*. So from the students' point of view, I think they really feel like there isn't anything" (emphasis added). Perez's statement makes it clear that, at his medical school, the lack of coherence and smattered curricular placement of the social sciences material rendered the content nearly inconsequential.

The smattering and invisibility that Perez pointed to were outcomes of the curricular designers' decisions. And decisions like these were most apparent in the curricular maps at medical schools, as featured in figures 3.1 and 3.2. Curricular maps reveal medical school leaders' decisions about how much time should be dedicated to a

Wk	Mn	Day	Mon	Tues	Wed	Thurs	Fri
Class of 2021							
1	Jul	31	2017–18		Orientation		
2	Aug	7	Genetics and Health (4 weeks)				
3		14					
4		21					
5		28					
6	Sep	5	Holiday				
7		11					
8		18					
9		25	Foundations of Medicine (12 weeks)				
10	Oct	2					
11		9					
12		16					
13		23					
14		30	Nutrition (1 week)				
15	Nov	6					Holiday
16		13	Foundations of Medicine				
17		20				Thanksgiving	
18		27					
19	Dec	4	Preceptorship (3 weeks)				
20		11					
21		18					
22		25	Holiday (2 weeks)				
23	Jan	1					
24		8	Health Policy (1 week)				
25		15	Fundamentals of Microbiology and Immunology (5 weeks)				
26		22					
27		29					
28	Feb	5					
29		12	Intro to Clinical Oncology (2 weeks)				
30		19					
31		26	Spring Break				
32	Mar	5	Respiratory Systems (4 weeks)				
33		12					
34		19					
35		26					
36	Apr	2					
37		9	Cardiovascular Systems (4 weeks)				
38		16					
39		23					
40		30					
41	May	7	Renal Systems (4 weeks)				
42		14					
43		21					
44		28	Preceptorship (1 week)				
45	Jun	4	Electives (7 weeks)				
46		11					
47		18					
48		25					
49	Jul	2					
50		9					
51		16					
52		23					

(Vertical labels, left section: Practice of Medicine; Research Practicum; Practice of Medicine)

Wk	Mn	Day	Mon	Tues	Wed	Thurs	Fri
1	Aug	13	Gastroenterology and Hepatology (5 weeks)				
2		20					
3		27					
4	Sep	4					
5		10					
6		17	Clinical Neuroscience (7 weeks)				
7		24					
8	Oct	1					
9		8					
10		15					
11		22					
12		29					
13	Nov	5	Preceptorship (1 week)				
14		13	Holiday	Pain and Addiction			
15		19					Thanksgiving
16		26	Dermatology and Musculoskeletal (4 weeks)				
17	Dec	3					
18		10					
19		17	Holiday (2 weeks)				
20		24					
21	Jan	2	Endocrinology and Reproduction (4 weeks)				
22		7					
23		14					
24		22					
25		28	Hematology (4 weeks)				
26	Feb	4					
27		11					
28		18					
29		25	NBME BSE and CSE				
30	Mar	4	Spring Break				
31		11	USMLE STEP 1 Study				
32		18					
33		25					
34	Apr	8					
35		15					
36		22					
37		29	Clerkship Orientation				
38	May	6	Clerkships				
39		13					
40		20					
41		27					
42	Jun	3					
43		10					
44		17					
45		24					
46	Jul	1					
47		8					
48		15					
49		22					
50		29					
51	Aug	5					
52		12					

(Vertical labels, right section: Practice of Medicine; Practice of Medicine)

FIGURE 3.1 Shoehorning the social sciences into the medical school curriculum in years 1 and 2

	August	September	October	November	December	January	February	March	April	May	June	July
Foundational Phase	Scientific Foundations I and Foundations of Patient Care		Exam Period I / Intersession I	Scientific Foundations II and Immunology, Rheumatology, Dermatology, and Infectious Diseases	Exam Period II / Break I / Intersession II	Cardiovascular, Renal, and Respiratory Systems		Exam Period III / Break II / Intersession III	Gastrointestinal, Reproductive, and Endocrine Systems		Exam Period IV / Break III	
	Longitudinal Courses Electives		OSCE I	Longitudinal Courses Electives	OSCE II	Longitudinal Courses Electives		OSCE III	Longitudinal Courses Electives		OSCE IV	
Core Clinical Phase	Musculoskeletal System, Hematology		Exam Period V / Intersession IV	Central Nervous System I and II	Exam Period VI / Break IV	Step I		e-Portfolio / Pathophysiology	Core Clinical Rotations		Intersession V / Break V	
	Longitudinal Courses Electives		OSCE V	Longitudinal Courses Hospital Visits	OSCE VI							
	Core Clinical Rotations				Break VI	Core Clinical Rotations		Intersession VI / e-Portfolio	Fourth-Year Activities			
Advanced Clinical Phase	Fourth-Year Activities				Break VII	Fourth-Year Activities		Graduation				

FIGURE 3.2 Shoehorning the social sciences into the medical school curriculum in years 1 to 4

particular topic, when it will be taught, the pedagogical format of instruction, and whether it should be required. They are snapshots of how the school enacts their UME curriculum in accordance with and reference to the required LCME standards and suggested humanities programming. After designing course maps, the course directors (may) decide what to teach each day and the time of instruction, as well as select who will lecture on what. At this point, the individual clinical faculty members slotted to give a particular lecture or facilitate a small group on a topic may have more say in how they teach whatever topic is on their plate.

Most medical schools' curricular designers shoehorned in the social sciences by placing these disciplines into small and awkward places. Figure 3.1 shows a typical medical school's interpretation of the LCME standards for the first two years. This school's curricular designers shoehorned the social sciences into what they refer to as "intersessions," like with the "Health Policy" course. These one-week intersessions received very little attention relative to the rest of the courses (e.g., "Genetics and Health," "Foundations of Medicine," "Fundamentals of Microbiology and Immunology," etc.). They were also scheduled right after students returned from their holiday break, which was a less emphasized part of the academic year.

Dr. Giannattasio, a white female clinical faculty member at a medical school, had a similar curricular design as the school whose curricular map is shown in figure 3.2. As the dean of UME, she explained: "[W]e structured our clerkship year in twelve-week blocks and between the twelve-week blocks they would do this one-week intersession. We'd visit cultural competency within that intersession." After she elaborated how students ran from their clerkship electives to rotations in neurology, pediatrics, and surgery at different hospitals, they came back for one week to take this intersession. She expressed that there just was not enough in place for students to learn much, saying, "[T]here's not much formal instruction . . . they're away doing electives and finishing up requirements." It was not just the timing of the intersessions in terms of breaks but also in terms of placement relative to the rest of the curriculum. The snapshot of all four years of UME is captured in figure 3.2, which shows the rotation-intersession-rotation curricular design.

As Dr. Perez mentioned and I can corroborate, most students described the amount of in-class, faculty-led time devoted to the social sciences and covering the prescriptive LCME standards as minimal—sometimes just half a day, other times a whole week, like at Dr. Giannattasio's school. Another example of the way the social sciences were shoehorned comes from a different school, where the "students explore how socio-economic disparities based on zip code, living conditions and access impact health in families. Students will reflect on their own biases and knowledge of the principles of bioethics as they apply them to case scenarios with family members." The entirety of this school's social sciences instruction (and bioethics) happened in *one single day* out of four years. In this school, the instruction was also done in an interprofessional setting, which made it seem like this skill set was not unique to being a physician and thus could have the effect of demoting its topical importance for medical students who want to learn what only physicians must know.[17]

While many schools would do a mixture of both approaches, as captured in figures 3.1 and 3.2, it is worth noting that curricular designers felt torn between independent and integrated models. The "Health Policy" course in figure 3.1 displays an independent course design, and the "Introduction to Clinical Medicine" course in the same figure shows an integrated one. As Dr. Sampson, a white female humanist, mentioned, "[I]t's really hard to figure out structures that are more compatible with the message that we're trying to convey. I think format is super important and really needs to be considered carefully." With the integrated model, the advantage was that students could get to learn this fundamental knowledge and the skills and have them reinforced by multiple instructors; the upside to independent courses was that students could build a deeper understanding through repeated and concentrated time on the topic. Running vertically in figure 3.1 is the "Introduction to Clinical Medicine" course, which was this school's version of a doctoring or POM course. In the associated course description for "Introduction to Clinical Medicine," the school says that the course covered "patient interviewing skills, professionalism and ethics, medical system structure and health disparities, cultural competency, provision of health maintenance and use of health guidelines."

The curricular designers commonly decided to teach the social sciences in courses like the "Introduction to Clinical Medicine" course, or POM course, which was a fateful choice guided by the *clinical witnessing* rationale. Because clinical witnessing is premised on seeing another's experience as a source of information, snippets of social science were often included as a part of "clinical skills" in the POM sequence rather than the "basic knowledge" blocks. The connection between clinical experience and POM instruction was exemplified by Dr. Johnson, a white female clinical faculty member, who said, "[T]he areas where the content is related to humanities and social sciences would be in our interviewing course . . . we would have a lecture on interviewing patients about sexuality or interviewing patients who don't speak English as their first language." Johnson continued, "[S]tudents also have a lot of experience from cases, specific cases. For example, they may be told, '[O]kay Mrs. Smith is coming in and is a standardized patient. And Mrs. Smith is Indian transgender.'" She paused for a moment and then went on to say to me that at their school, they "give [students] a *complex* case, a *complex* individual. That contextualizes, I think, for students and makes it clinically relevant. Do you know what I'm saying?"

Filtered through her clinical witnessing perspective, Johnson's hypothetical case married the best intentions with the worst social science. Under the clinical witnessing rationale that curricular designers invoked, it seemed perfectly legitimate to engage in these cases. Clinical faculty members had little understanding about the epistemic implications of placing the content on the social sciences as part of the "interviewing skills" section of UME or for locating the source of "complexity" on the individual nonwhite, non-cisgender patient. But their decisions to place the social sciences in the POM course had the effect of placing that material in the realm of experience rather than knowledge. As Johnson's hypothetical case illustrated, by choosing "Mrs. Smith is Indian transgender" as the exemplary case, she showed *who* the profession deemed as "socially complex," thus creating the conditions under which clinical faculty members could exoticize and pathologize socially marginalized groups.[18] The mere existence of the term "socially complex" implies who the profession thinks is "socially straightforward."[19]

I will return to the content-related failures encapsulated in these examples in the next chapter, but for the purpose of this chapter, I would like to focus on the decisions that the clinical faculty members made regarding curricular design. With independent courses, the average amount of time spent on social sciences within my sample of medical school curricula was just one week out of forty to forty-six weeks during which students take coursework, or just over 2 percent of curricular time in a given academic year. Thus, in many ways, the shoehorning of social sciences into one week appeared to render this material merely symbolic. But the curricular practices were quite productive and ideological. They did more than simply nothing because these decisions about curricular practices were not neutral. Johnson's hypothetical case illustrates how these decisions contributed to the medical student's epistemic socialization and reinforced white cisgender norms. Curricular designers thus contributed to the marginalization of social scientific content with their top-down decisions about where, when, and for how long the LCME standards were taught at their medical schools.

INCLUSION AS ADMISSIONS

Detailing the curricular designers' decision making vis-à-vis the LCME standards and the social sciences was relatively straightforward in comparison to the other curricular decisions that clinical faculty members made. Another, more subtle way that the curricular designers included the social sciences was through admissions. They also did this with the humanities. Regarding the social sciences, *inclusion-as-admissions* came up through the clinical faculty members' valuation of diversity for the POM small groups. Dr. Giannattasio, introduced earlier in this chapter, was going into more detail about how her school planned to engage in the instruction of social sciences in lieu of "formal instruction" that they would not have during those intersessions. She described the following exercise: "I mean we did one of these exercises where you like all stand up, and then you sit down after the certain qualifiers and you see who's left standing."

This exercise prompted students to identify publicly with particular social backgrounds (e.g., sit down if you have never experienced racial discrimination), and then used it as a springboard for specific discussions around social categories like gender identity and race (e.g., those left standing, please share).

Another medical school's course description boasted, "the half-day, off-campus session utilizes experiential exercises and small group discussions to give first year medical students an opportunity to learn about different populations they will serve and to explore ways to communicate in cross-cultural situations." At a session I observed at the AAMC annual meeting on medical education, panelists shared this same exercise for teaching social sciences, calling it the "standing for" activity. In that same session, another panelist said that these POM small groups were a good setting for students to learn this material because "students know more than faculty." While I will return to that latter point in the next chapter, what is important here is that admissions seemed to be the key piece of the curricular practices puzzle for the clinical faculty members in charge of curricular design at these schools.

With these types of "standing for" exercises, students with visible social identities, like race, are conscripted into participating based solely on their membership in that particular social group. I call this practice the *conscripted curriculum*, in which educators rely on students to teach each other from their experiences as members of social groups. The clinical faculty members I spoke with—both in their capacities as curricular designers and implementers—explained to me that students marked as "diverse"—as in, nonwhite, nonelite, nonheteronormative—brought experiences to the POM course and that these experiences formed the content of the instruction of race, gender, and sexuality. Dr. Glynn, a white female UME dean, elaborated further on the notion that student-led sharing of diverse experiences was a way for students to fulfill the LCME standards when she explained to me: "So, it's a really hard thing to teach but we have a very diverse group of students in the class from a lot of backgrounds. Purposely. There are men, women purposely drawn from all different racial, ethnic, and religious backgrounds, transgender, even people from Iraq that are princes, just a lot of people. They're coming from very different backgrounds." The inclusion-as-admissions approach was evident with Glynn's usage of "purposely," which was also invoked by Dr. George, a white male clinical faculty member at another school who said, "[W]e have small groups that meet over two years and they are more—we purposely mix our groups so that we have a mixture of male, female, different races, ages." Curricular designers like Glynn and George viewed racial and gender diversity of their matriculants as part of their strategy for meeting their professional curricular requirements.

In addition, Dr. Kerns, a white male clinical faculty member and course director of the POM sequence where social science was taught at his school, said that the reason why the instruction was effective was because they were "a pretty diverse student body so it's not like there wouldn't be a wealth of *experience* in the room." In response to my question about when students learn about race, Dr. Lombard, a white female clinical faculty member, pointed out that "some students, they're not native English speakers or from America, so they have their own cultural concepts that they bring to the patient and the case, so I think that's where students get the content." Dr. Stephens, a white male clinical faculty member, claimed that the small group was beneficial as a space to learn about social sciences because it was a supportive environment; he continued, telling me that "something that's very helpful to us in this is that our student body is actually quite diverse." When I asked Robby, a white medical student, how he had learned about social inequalities, he mentioned his fellow students. He said, "I think the thing that pushes students to think about it more is other students. And I don't think it necessarily should be the responsibility of the rest of the class to educate their classmates, but I think that's what happens because of class structure." Robby highlighted how other students were educating their peers, and that this was part of the class *structure*. It was part of the curricular design. While this pedagogical approach might befuddle a social scientist, it is logically consistent with the epistemic filter that accompanies clinical witnessing. As with the case-learning method that Johnson described, with the conscripted curriculum, the clinical faculty members are making curricular decisions that foreground experience as central to learning about social inequalities. In this way, the inclusion-as-admissions approach operates in a way that is similar to what Derrick Bell described as "interest convergence," where white clinical faculty members support the inclusion of more marginalized students so that they can teach their peers. Such a curricular practice is reminiscent of the "diversity bargain" that white Harvard students made in valuing a "diverse" cohort in Natasha Warikoo's research on higher education.[20] With the diversity bargain, the white students were accepting of a more diverse student body if those nonwhite students provided them with personal gains, like learning about different cultures in their diverse classrooms. The white clinical faculty members also seem to value admitting nonwhite students for what they could bring to the classroom and designed the curricular practices around that premise.

The inclusion-as-admissions approach also occurred with the humanities, which I will introduce with an extended example. In a 2015 publication in *Columbia Magazine* about concert-level musicians attending Columbia University's medical school, the author asked: "So how did all these concert-level musicians end up at [the school]? Last year, of some 7,800 applicants, the school enrolled 160 future doctors, more than a third of whom were as comfortable with operettas as operations."[21] The piece, with its clever alliterations, went on to focus on particular students and to describe their interview process. One such student, Harvard-trained and Broadway-honed Jessica Means, had an admissions interview that was "less medicine than Mendelssohn, less pleurisy than Debussy. She remarked how, during her interview, she was struck by her interviewer's interest in music, saying: "[W]e didn't talk about medicine at all. He wanted to know everything about music. He thought it was wonderful . . . It blows my mind how talented these people are . . . Musical Monday is conservatory level.'"[22] Musical Mondays at this medical school allowed students to engage in humanities activities—similarly to social sciences, what was key was that the admitted students were the ones bringing the content. They were not learning anything with this programming beyond what the students brought to the table.

In answering the question about why they admit so many concert musicians, the director of admissions at Columbia University's medical school, Stephen Nicholas, said in this article: "We have one highest desire: to find people who will make great doctors. The question facing all medical schools is, 'How do you find those individuals?' Some schools use metrics; some look at undergraduate majors. Those things are important, but they're not what make this place tick. We think there are a lot of *surrogate* measures." Reminiscent of Dr. Carlyle Jacobsen's remarks in chapter 1 and the inclusion-as-admissions approach that helped build the U.S. medical profession in the mid-twentieth century, contemporary medical schools still seem to value what "conservatory level" musical abilities signify. Given the material and temporal commitment necessary to do these pursuits well, students from these well-heeled elite backgrounds are more likely to be these people.[23]

Medical students and educators in my sample also spoke of the "conservatory-level" abilities of many medical students. One white female medical student, Joan, explained that "there were cultural performances, like I had a friend sing Italian opera." Another Latina medical student, Jennifer, told me how they "had a talent show at the end of second year. What was interesting was that the talent show was really amazing because you'd have these people who would bounce in and they'd be like, 'hey you know I had been playing piano since I was two,' or 'I'm a professional this and professional that.' They'd put together some of these performances with classmates that was pretty breathtaking." Jennifer touched on how effortlessly these talents were put on display, noting how they would "bounce in" and casually announce their lifelong immersion in a particular humanities field. "Professional this and professional that" further encapsulates how these forms of expertise were perceived as effortless, a point I will return to in chapter 5.

Just as students are competing for admissions spots, medical schools are in competition for the best and brightest students. Given the escalation of requirements for getting into medical school, as I discussed in chapter 2, possessing expertise in the humanities was seen as a mark of distinction, and medical schools wanted to cater to those sensibilities in their students upon their arrival. As a result, some of the schools often discussed their humanities programming—even if, as conceptualized here, they were a far cry from the critical potential captured in the Fundamental Role of Arts and Humanities in Medical Education (FRAHME) report's curricular dreams—as a draw for students to continue cultivating their interests in the context of the medical school that was seen as "intellectually deadening." Schools, like the one where white male humanist Dr. Williams taught, deliberately recruited students "who were going to be more well rounded, more humanistically focused, more creative types—and that would eventually parlay into having a different kind of culture in the medical school and different kinds of physicians." Some educators even noted that "some of our better students came because of the medical humanities program," as Dr. Morris, a white male humanist, did. White male medical student John said his medical school was "very pro humanities," noting that his school boasted often how "30 percent of us were some sort of humanities or social science majors."

More than simply attracting the "best" students, some educators described humanities expertise as giving students a competitive edge in gaining prestigious residency spots—showing how the profession valued this "surrogate" measure every step along the professionalization pipeline. Dr. Geronimos, a white female social scientist who ran the nonbiomedical programming at her medical school, said, "[If students] are thinking about looking ahead to a residency at some place competitive, having this degree really helps their residency applications and will be discussed in their Dean's letter." The "degree" that Geronimos was referring to was that some students can pursue "scholarly concentrations" as a way to highlight their immersion in the humanities disciplines. Another medical school's course description of a humanities course noted, "[O]nce a semester, students write a Signature Reflection, which is stored in the student's portfolio and available as a point of reference when the students begin to apply to residency programs." Because there were no humanities requirements—just profession-wide programming suggestions—the curricular designers have even more leeway in their interpretive decisions around how to incorporate these fields.

Musical Mondays would be nothing without the student musicians. POM courses would be lacking in content without the students from socially marginalized backgrounds. Thus, in addition to shoehorning in the social sciences, curricular designers also included the social sciences—and humanities—via admissions. This approach both obviated the need for faculty and emphasized an understanding of a revered social identity (white elite people) and an othered one (nonwhite, nonelite people), a point to which I will return in chapter 4 when I discuss the implementation of these curricular practices in the classroom.

OFFERING THE HUMANITIES AS ELECTIVES

The talent show that revealed the inclusion-as-admissions approach was indicative of a much larger strategy that curricular designers took when including the humanities into UME: embracing the flexibility of the humanities and leaning into their status as electives.

TABLE 3.1 COURSE TITLES OF HUMANITIES ELECTIVES

"Medical History and Humanities"	"Short History of Medicine"
"Surgery Throughout the Ages"	"Self and Culture"
"The Healer's Art"™	"Visual Thinking at the Art Gallery"
"Creative Writing"	"Medical Cineforum"
"HeART Stories: Building Empathy Through the Arts"	"Culinary Medicine"
"The Language of Music: Improvisation in Sound"	"Science Fiction and Medicine"
"When Doctors Become Patients"	"Graphic Medicine"
"Psychiatry at the Movies"	"Theater and the Experience of Illness"
"Humanities and Medicine"	"Jazz and the Art of Storytelling"
"Major Religious Traditions"	"Patient, Physician, and Drama"
"Dissecting to Think: History of Anatomy"	"Literature and Medicine"
"Doctors on Film"	"Art and Medicine"

Clinical faculty members, in their capacities as curricular designers, were not focused on accreditation with the humanities but rather on addressing the empathy problem that they also experienced in their clinical work. Including the humanities as electives was a choice, and three features to the elective structure were key: the flexibility in content and delivery, the juxtaposition of the elective and the required coursework (perhaps captured by the *extra*curricular nature of the elective), and the devolution of responsibility to the student to elect to take the course. These electives took on forms such as book clubs, art discussions, affinity groups, and talent shows and might draw from art, music, literature, or even comics. See table 3.1 for a sample of some elective course titles.

Similar to the shoehorned incorporation of the social sciences, the humanities electives did not occupy a lot of curricular time.

With these curricular practices, the educators were less concerned with the humanities disciplines themselves; they were also not interested in rigorous or critical study. One school stated on their course website that they offered extracurricular engagements with humanities, known as "enrichment activities," where the academic program included: "reading and discussion with clinical faculty, special theater events, museum visits, and films."

An example of how a common humanities elective was described is "The Healer's Art"™, which is a branded and commodified course that many medical schools offer. According to Rachel Naomi Remen, the white female clinical faculty member who created "The Healer's Art"™, it was offered at 50 percent of U.S. medical schools at the time of my data collection.[24] One school that adopted the course described the elective as follows:

> Learning how to preserve and strengthen your own humanity, your sense of the physician's work, and your ability to handle loss and remain open-hearted may make the difference between professional burnout and a rich and fulfilling life. In Healer's Art™, we will be talking about meaning and service, sharing loss, finding healing, strengthening our personal commitment and uncovering the spiritual dimensions of the practice of medicine for ourselves. Meetings are held in the evenings at an off-campus site, most likely at a manor which has a great setting that will remind you of Clue. This is an elective class, and you WILL enjoy it if you take it. There are no quizzes and no presentations.

There was a lot to unpack in this course description, from the fact that it was a commodified course to the rejoinder to students that "You WILL enjoy it if you take it," containing an ironic air of compulsory enjoyment. The structure of the course was also highlighted: off campus, in the evening, elective, no homework; it was emphatically for fun.

The course description's overall tone was emblematic of the unbridled positivity about the humanities that I kept encountering during my research, from the AAMC panels to interviews with clinical faculty members about the humanities. The humanities seemed to be ubiquitously celebrated and adored; they were incorporated in an almost kitschy manner, like a "Keep Calm and Take a Humanities Elective" mug. The clinical faculty members I spoke to and observed seemed to believe that students truly loved these electives that they categorized as humanities. Medical schools spotlighted them in materials advertising their programs to prospective students, no matter how little time was actually dedicated to these humanities-based electives, for example, a half-day workshop featuring a "mindfulness retreat, figure sculpture, medical illustration, horsemanship and medicine, improvisational acting, improvisational music, music and dance, yoga, journalism, writing and medicine, photography, poetry, among others." While I will delve deeper into the content in the next chapter, for now I want to highlight this school's curricular designers' decision to have the entirety of their humanities content in a half-day session.

Although this was a half-day activity that happened once a year, the medical school deemed it attractive enough to prospective students that they included it on their list of course offerings and programming for students to see—whether to recruit talented humanists or to portray itself as an enticing place for those who also wanted fun. With that latter point, and as The Healer's Art™ course description suggested, the humanities were a break, with enjoyment guaranteed. The majority of clinical faculty members and students articulated the perceived goals for including the humanities in their UME curriculum in this narrow, therapeutically utilitarian manner. Students were so primed for this therapeutic appreciation that they went into these electives expecting cathartic outcomes. For example, the first time that he taught a "Literature in Medicine" elective, Dr. Donovan, a white male humanist, laughed when he recalled how he thought, "I'm going to transform your lives." When he got the postclass evaluations, he was "expecting these very earth-shattering things" but then he realized that "the majority of people just said it was really relaxing, it was a really great break from anatomy or something." The people that Donovan was referring to were clinical faculty members and medical students because the elective was open to anyone along the physician pipeline. Donovan's experience teaching this course pointed to one of the central ways in which the humanities were designed in UME: as therapeutic curricular practices.

The humanities thus were conceptualized by the clinical faculty curricular designers to help address one of the most pressing parts of the empathy problem facing the medical profession: burnout. Recall from chapter 2 that fifty-six of ninety respondents brought up burnout in response to my question about whether they taught the humanities. Making the link explicit between burnout and humanities was Dr. Busler, a white female humanist who described a literature in medicine group at her school as a space for the physicians and students to meet and receive support. When I asked whether they had any humanities offerings for her students, she said, "[W]e have groups that meet every week. Some groups meet once a month for forty-five minutes. It's really a professional development group and can be very helpful to, you know, provide support for the group members and be a way to lessen burnout, I think. We do it really as an offering and as a kind of supportive resource." Busler renamed the course to capture more accurately what she felt was happening there—it was a burnout support group.

Humanities, conceptualized in this way, allowed students to improve their well-being so that medical care could also be improved. I asked Dr. Brooks, a white male clinical faculty member who led the literature in medicine group at his school, about the value of reading literature for physicians. He explained: "I think it does decrease burnout. I think that coming out of that rigorous scientific approach and being in a place where you're not graded, where you're not asked to come up with the right answer, where you're just asking them to really think about different scenarios up close and talk through it with other people and bounce off their ideas, consider their points of view, I think that's the value." Brooks's comments illustrated yet another way in which the particular strengths of the humanities as therapeutic—not graded, no right or wrong answer, just bouncing off ideas—were put to work to combat the empathy problem. It was also a place in the curriculum where people were not asked to think, which would incense any card-carrying humanist.

With this approach to incorporation, clinical faculty members conceptualized the humanities as a set of protective meaning-making tools that would give (future) physicians the sensibilities needed to survive in a health-care setting brimming with causes of burnout, causes such as a lack of resources, "socially complex" patients (as clinical faculty members liked to say), stressful work conditions, and perceived low pay. Just as the basic sciences served as a scapegoat for the issues plaguing the inclusion of the social sciences, biomedicine served as this looming, dehumanizing, boogeyman that the humanities could help students better cope with. In this sense, these humanities electives serve as examples of how the humanities are *used* by—in service of reinforcing the status quo of—the medical profession. The humanities were applied to achieve certain ends: a fun, stress-relieving break from the real work involving biomedical knowledge.

Because these curricular practices were created in response to the burnout crisis, requiring students to put in a lot of work when engaging with the humanities seems antithetical to its objectives. If educators justify including the humanities as therapeutic by convincing students and administrators that such electives help address burnout, then a consequence is that educators cannot require students to put in a lot of work learning the particulars of the humanities. They are also not having students encounter critical or upsetting work about the medical profession or health—which is at odds with some of the profession-wide stated goals regarding the humanities as captured by the FRAHME initiative. I want to emphasize how the flexibility of these humanities electives allows the leaders of medical schools to address crises, like burnout, and not disrupt the fragile haphazard organization of curricular design.

* * *

In this chapter, I have shown how the disorganization of medical schools and subsequent dominance of clinical faculty members create the conditions under which professional curricular guidelines were interpreted through the filter of clinical experience. They shoehorned in the social sciences, relied on students to "bring the content" of the social sciences and humanities, and transformed the humanities into therapeutic electives. When curricular designers made decisions about what, how, and when to include the humanities and social sciences, they capitalized on the flexibility of curricular practices and designed courses that reinforce the status quo (white, elite, cisgender, clinical). Clinical faculty members justified the inclusion of social sciences based on clinical relevance, but because of the epistemic limitations of this clinical witnessing justification, they did not know how to teach the critical and structural lessons that these fields could impart. In fact, clinical faculty members' reliance on students to teach each other from their experiences underscores their own lack of expertise.[25] It is precisely the capacities and choices of individual faculty members as they enact the curricular practices designed by their specific medical school that will be the focus of the next chapter.

4

ENACTING CURRICULAR PRACTICES IN THE CLASSROOM

Given the decisions made by the curricular designers at each medical school, much of the context for curricular injustice was set before students encountered the content in the classroom. To introduce the forms of failure that occurred in the context of everyday instruction, I will introduce Sam, a white female medical student. During our discussion, Sam recounted this "awkward" memory of a clinical faculty member trying to facilitate a conversation in their practice of medicine (POM) small group. Sam told me that the white male clinical faculty member started the lesson by describing a hypothetical clinical case: "Okay you have a patient who needs to lose weight with diabetes or whatever and you want to go over different foods that they can eat . . . He goes, '[W]ell you can't just tell them to cut out carbs because they're eating, like, fajita bread and this is their normal diet . . . so you have to work with them.'" As she was telling the story, Sam kept pausing to double-down on the awkwardness of this pedagogical scene. She noted how the clinical faculty member's inability to utilize the appropriate term of "tortilla" and instead using "fajita bread" underscored the poor delivery and cultural stereotyping. Sam went on to recount another example from this educator's facilitation: "I remember that as one example of the Hispanic population, we watched a video and a lady's crying because she can't get enchiladas. You feel awkward for watching." This awkward moment was the only time Sam could remember learning about the Liaison Committee on Medical Education (LCME) Standard 7 on social sciences.

With regard to the humanities, Gyi, a South Asian male medical student, took a "Literature in Medicine" elective at his school because he wanted to engage with the humanities. When I asked what kinds of books he read, he demurred, saying that the way his clinical faculty member led the course, it was "essentially group therapy." Clinical faculty members and students alike often offered accounts of how humanities operated in the classroom—as tools or spaces that allowed medical students and faculty to relax and enjoy one another's company; play with something fun; and contemplate how the book, art, or music made them feel. The humanities, when implemented by clinical faculty members, were transformed into a "social, a nice stress relief kind of thing." They were therapeutic curricular practices rather than critical ones.

These examples from Sam's and Gyi's experiences with their required and elective courses are revealing in a couple of ways. First, and perhaps most vividly, in using the passive language of "awkward"—rather than calling the clinical faculty member's example what it was, which was racist[1]—Sam was showing the fruits of her facilitator's educational labor. She did not have the language for or awareness around racism. Gyi also did not have a takeaway from the humanities elective beyond it being therapeutic. While student reception will be the focus of chapter 5, the second point this example from Sam in particular elicits is the broader issue with (mostly white, mostly clinical) medical educators in the classroom: they lack expertise. As Sam's clinical faculty member's use of the term "fajita bread" demonstrates, clinical faculty members' limited understandings produce curricular practices that diverge from the curricular dreams of critical and reflexive doctoring. Not only do they fail to address the LCME standards and the equity problems undergirding them, but they do so in ways that reify social inequalities.

While clinical faculty members lacked social scientific and humanistic expertise, they had an abundance of clinical expertise, which patterned their approach to enacting curricular practices in the classroom. Via their *clinical witnessing*, clinical faculty members valued patient cases and lived experience rather than systematically researched bodies of knowledge, thus affecting how the social sciences were taught in the classroom. And by centering their own experiences with the difficulties of their clinical work, clinical faculty members viewed the humanities as tools to help them cope with their jobs. In both cases—social sciences and humanities—clinical experience served as a proxy for social sciences and humanities expertise. And in both cases, there were significant consequences for how curricular practices were enacted in the classroom: as I will show, the central curricular injustices occurring with in-classroom instruction were curricular practices that were inaccurate, placating, and inequitable.

CLINICAL FACULTY MEMBERS' LIMITED EXPERTISE

As described in chapter 3, the decisions made by the curricular designers constrained the incorporation of the social scientific and humanistic lessons contained in the profession-wide curricular dreams. And while I have already been detailing the clinical faculty members' lack of expertise, here I want to go into more detail about how it emanated and operated, ultimately capturing the mismatch between clinical faculty members' well-intentioned desires to address the equity and empathy problems but their lack of capacity to do so. One South Asian male clinical faculty member, Dr. Gupta, articulated this mismatch between desire and capacity by commenting at first how "the LCME requirements—they tell us we need to be able to recognize biases in ourselves, others, and health-care delivery. They tell us we need to be professional." Then he went to assert that, at his school, "we could use anthropology, history, or sociology to teach this . . . the idea would be that we would have one trained facilitator for every ten students." He then lamented the curricular approach at his school, remarking with an eyeroll, "[B]ut in reality we have 800 students and ask them to reflect on 'professionalism.'" As Gupta emphasized, his school would ideally employ trained experts to instruct students on the social scientific material, but it does not.

Dr. Pultz, a white female social scientist at another medical school, told me about how dire some of the humanities instruction was at their school. She explained that, to pull off a seminar where students critically interrogated the medical profession, they would need to have the "luxury" of hiring "real historians." She said, "[Y]ou know, we're not like [elite school]; we don't have PhDs who can teach all this stuff." Pultz also drew attention to the mismatch between intellectual needs and personnel. At the schools where Gupta and Pultz work, they simply did not have the *intellectual infrastructure* to support these curricular dreams, whereby intellectual infrastructure captures an organization's personnel, time, and resources necessary to accomplish the knowledge-related task they seek to accomplish.

As a result of the decisions medical school leaders made about hiring, where they relied on part-time and volunteer labor, clinical faculty members were the ones who engaged in the day-to-day instruction in the classroom, as was often the case with curricular design. Dr. Krebs, a white male clinical faculty member, described his school's approach to electives as "variable depending on the presentation, depending on the course. We have [a] collection of emeritus faculty who have an interest to teach history." Curricular designers at medical schools used these clinical faculty members because they were volunteering their time, and these electives could thus operate at no cost, especially if they were held off campus in an educator's home. Another white female clinical faculty member, Dr. Robinson, described how their medical school relied on the generosity of the clinical faculty members, saying that some of their electives could go away because the clinical faculty members who were running their art and medicine meetup group no longer wanted to foot the "pizza bill." Relying on the clinical faculty members' generosity translates to their control, as white male humanist, Dr. Mayberry, noted, expressing that "some of the courses have take-home reading and some don't. It's really up to the instructors. And the courses really vary a lot in structure. Some of them are very involved and meet twelve times in a semester; some of them meet four times and that's the whole course."

Even with professional guidelines and materials, the clinical faculty members delivering the content still had a tremendous amount of interpretive leeway. For example, Dr. Harrison, a white male humanist who worked in the POM sequence at his medical school, elaborated on the interpretive power of clinical faculty members, saying, "There's always sort of a guide and so it's like cover these cases, answer these questions, have an open conversation about these things. And some people just want to follow that sort of diligently, others less so. I don't think the students get sort of a uniform experience across their small group." At Harrison's medical school, the clinical faculty members lectured or facilitated based on notes or slides that they did not personally develop—the course directors or undergraduate medical education (UME) committee did. As Dr. Watkins, a white male clinical faculty member, pointed out to me, this form of faculty inexperience could manifest where, "depending on who the lecturer is, he or she may not be—they may not know anything about environmental factors. So sometimes the lecturer may say, 'I'm really not sure; I've not heard that.'" Both Harrison and Watkins highlighted that, despite the potential for oversight, there was additional interpretative slippage.

Students brought up this inexperience, too. Students often remarked on their clinical faculty members' lack of expertise, like Sam did in the introduction to this chapter when she described how "awkward" her POM facilitator was. Andrew, a white male medical student, explained to me when I asked him about his "Art in Medicine" elective, "[I]t is different every time . . . I tried to pin it down, it was like, what is this series? And it didn't make sense because it was kind of like whatever." Like Gyi, who had "group therapy" as the takeaway from the "Literature and Medicine" course, Andrew could not pinpoint a specific humanities-related lesson from the clinical faculty course facilitators. Jeremy, a white male student, simply laughed when I asked about how instruction of social sciences occurred at his school. He commented more explicitly how the clinical faculty members at his school were "not equipped to teach anthropology or sociology."

Dr. Mogin, a white male social scientist who taught at a medical school, observed how it took a certain skill set to be able to teach the social science content, saying, rhetorically, "[W]hat we're talking about is sort of taking on the multi-headed monster of racism, right?" He continued with the monster metaphor, articulating how "the head of the monster shows itself in health care and health access and well-being of people. So at some point we have to have some very tough conversations about power and race and racism—and to be able to engage in and facilitate those conversations is pretty high-level skill, right?" Despite Mogin's point, most medical schools deputized clinical faculty members with this instruction rather than hiring social scientists to design—let alone teach—this content. Medical educators, across rank, social background, and disciplinary training, all bemoaned the state of faculty development for clinical faculty members.

To illustrate these faculty development woes, I draw on an interview I had with Dr. Bennett, a Black female clinical faculty member and dean of diversity, equity, and inclusion at a medical school and a former POM course director. She described a two-hour faculty training that she did for the POM clinical faculty. Bennett gave the participants a worksheet with seven social categories on it (i.e., age, gender, sexual orientation, race, ethnicity, disability, and class). Their instructions were to examine quickly their own biases around these social categories and rate their discomfort with the topic. She recounted:

When we debriefed about that worksheet it was fascinating that everyone skipped over sexual orientation and race. People did not want to have conversations about their own comfort or discomfort around issues of how they view people who are gay, and they didn't want to talk about how they viewed people who were racially different from them. They were really focused on issues of weight. So every person in the room wanted us to constantly talk about their discomfort with obese people.

While she discussed her reasons why the fixation on obesity was problematic in and of itself, Bennett went on to say how she tried to prompt the faculty to get someone—anyone—to discuss their level of comfort talking about sexual orientation or race.

She said that "everyone was like—oh yeah, we're good. They just didn't want to touch it." When she pushed it further, asking them if they found anything during the worksheet exercise that they were surprised about, she still got no engagement. She concluded, "And I'm a facilitator; I'm not forcing people. I was hoping someone would say something. Nah, nobody. They weren't telling. And I had like seventy-five faculty members there." If these seventy-five clinical faculty members were not able to discuss race or sexual orientation in a faculty workshop, they were certainly not equipped to discuss these topics in small groups with medical students. In addition, this training demonstrated to faculty members how to engage in the *conscripted curriculum*, described in chapter 3, albeit not effectively. Rather than receive instruction on systematically collected social scientific data about historical and contemporary manifestations of racism or heteronormativity, clinical faculty members were prompted to discuss their own feelings and experiences.

The faculty members in Bennett's workshop were like many of the clinical faculty members in the POM sequence, which was one of the main settings in which curricular designers decided to teach these social sciences subjects. At the Association of American Medical Colleges (AAMC) annual meetings, I often observed medical educators discussing how the clinical faculty members at their school had "no language to discuss race or LGBT in a sophisticated way." I also saw some clinical faculty members struggling with the complexity of social scientific concepts firsthand. At one session, where audience members were asked to answer a quiz about what they knew about social sciences concepts with fellow participants at their table, one participant said that they had "a hard time with big words" and then another chimed in saying that we should "answer the questions with the test-taking skills" we had, like process of elimination or marking one of several answer choices. The participants at the table ended up putting B for their answers rather than even trying. Clinical faculty members had both limited understandings and limited faculty development to augment those understandings.

The clinical faculty members had actively or passively accepted that they were doing their role without the necessary expertise. Teaching without qualifications is wild: imagine the roles being reversed and I were to teach anatomy at a medical school. Just the thought of that makes me anxious. But physicians doing social sciences? How hard could it be? Clinical faculty members often explicitly dismissed social sciences or humanities expertise by saying things like "anyone can teach it" or "I'm all good" in their faculty development. I also had countless interactions with clinical faculty members while doing my interviews where they were telling me about my own field. Perhaps this was Hippocratic hubris at work but it felt as if they did not need any more information because they saw and experienced it all in the clinic.

Social scientists and humanists who worked in medical schools were frustrated with the lack of clinical faculty expertise, particularly around an in-depth understanding of the critical lessons that the social sciences and humanities disciplines had to offer. For example, Dr. Grossmith, a white female social scientist at a medical school, told me about how there may have been "lots and lots of faculty development on bias, [but] when you suggest talking about scientific knowledge it's a much harder sell." As Bennett's example of a workshop on individual-level bias shows, even those faculty development workshops can fail, but Grossmith also pointed to how the content

itself was a big part of that failure. To correct that, she had been trying to encourage clinical faculty members to examine critically the
racist ideas embedded in the fundamental knowledge blocks on different organ systems and found that "no matter how delicately you
try to do it, it causes friction." Clinical faculty members at her school
were unable to interrogate their own knowledge base, and Grossmith
thought that "faculty development is something that I don't think
we've done as good a job as we need to, and I don't think anybody's
done as good a job." During our conversation, Grossmith talked about
how most medical schools lacked substantive faculty development
and that the "average medical school" served as "an example of when
you have a sprinkling of the social, but it's a *safe* social." For her clinical faculty colleagues, individual bias was safe; racism institutionalized
into medical knowledge was not. As one white male clinical faculty
member and dean of medical education, Dr. Capraro, explained, they
did "not have so much on racism," because "their focus in [their] curriculum tends to be on identifying those things that every medical
student should know . . . there are elements that could probably make
them a better physician but they aren't essential for every physician."
Knowing about racism was not "essential" for clinical care.

Most of the social sciences and humanities scholars who taught
at medical schools lamented the "shallow" or "introductory" understandings of their topics within the medical school and the constraint
that clinical faculty members' lack of expertise posed. Dr. Rogers, a
white male humanist, said that he was adept at what he called "code
switching," where he had to know when he had to "be explicit" about
the purpose of the humanities for medicine or when he could have
his "full literary hat on."[2] He thought it was a by-product of interdisciplinary collaboration itself, which forced a watering down of each
field being brought into conversation; the multiple perspectives "need
a lowest common denominator." Rogers elaborated further: "[Y]ou
have to have the ability to expand and collapse sometimes . . . and
it's not a compromise more so than it is an adjustment to make the

subject more palatable." In making the social sciences or humanities "more palatable" for clinical practice, the content took a hit. The clinical faculty members decontextualized and devalued the social sciences, and they transformed the humanities into interpersonal tools for placation.

DECONTEXTUALIZED AND DEVALUED SOCIAL SCIENCES

"The content is rough," the white male medical student, Jeremy, from earlier in this chapter, said of his school's instruction on social sciences. Because the LCME standards and the curricular practices of each medical school were simultaneously prescriptive and ambiguous, clinical faculty members had to interpret and then implement these curricular requirements in the classroom. The curricular designers shoehorned in the social sciences into one-week intersessions or the POM skills sequence, but clinical faculty members in the classroom also delimited its scope in terms of *what* social science was presented—and what was left out. They engaged in a range of curricular practices that contributed to the marginalization of the social sciences, consequential decisions because these curricular practices either did not address—or, worse, propagated additional—social inequalities.

Many medical schools limited the scope of their social scientific content on social inequalities to positivistic presentations about social groups. Presented as "just the facts" devoid of the historical and social context, these descriptions of social groups also tended to use biological or culturalist conceptualizations of human difference, akin to the "Hispanic woman is crying because she can't eat enchiladas" example that Sam discussed earlier in this chapter. She also said that they received "little snippets of documentaries . . . they had talked about migrant workers that are in different parts of the country, their experience and their health issues that are related to it." In addition to the content from these lectures or documentaries, the clinical faculty members upheld the value of lived experience as a source of social scientific knowledge, which, when understood in relation to the rest of the curriculum, devalued social science as merely anecdotal. In most cases, clinical faculty members did not engage in any instruction on constructionist or structural critiques of social inequalities and the medical profession.

In my discussion with Dr. Gattinella, a white social scientist, about how race and racism were addressed at his school, he said that, when it comes to the way the social scientific subjects and LCME standards were taught, his school used "the cultural competency frameworks around 'this group likes bananas and this group likes strawberries and this group likes cherries.'" He confessed that he found "that stuff an ache and that's what we were doing in our curriculum when I got here. There are a lot of people who like that stuff." Gattinella was frustrated that clinical faculty members at his school were teaching culturally reductive approaches to social differences, but he was right in that this approach had been popular. While there was—and continues to be—a robust movement underway to correct this from those promoting structural competency frameworks[3], the state of medical education was still mostly in the bananas, strawberries, and cherries phase when I carried out my research. As Gattinella concluded, "[T]his just does not reflect accurately what the social scientists say." The clinical faculty members were teaching inaccurate social science.

Typical of the clinical faculty members—and attendant curricular practices—that Gattinella spoke about is Dr. Bernansky, a white male course director at a medical school, who responded to my question about whether they taught the social sciences to their medical students by saying, "[S]o there's no specific area on nor titled that." He went on to explain that "within the POM curriculum we certainly do touch on those areas, it's like, in African American populations, prostate cancer would be far more prevalent, or in the LGBT community, one would have to be a little careful because the prevalence of this particular disease is more prevalent in this community than that community." Other clinical faculty members described similar limited, decontextualized approaches. Dr. Walcker, a white female clinical faculty member, explained to me that there was no specific course on the social sciences. When asked what they taught, she said: "I don't think so. I'm trying to think. I don't think there's a specific—I mean we talk about sort of the demographics of the patients." Walcker's example helps show both the lack of fluency with social sciences and the positivistic presentation of decontextualized statistics.

Dr. Jaffe, a white female clinical faculty member, said that their POM course "touches on epidemiology and quality improvement and systems change; so they have a bunch of sessions about social determinants of health." Dr. Tortora, a white male clinical faculty member at another school, noted that they cover implicit bias, disparities, and access to health care in their curricular intersessions. These examples epitomize how social sciences were delimited to these positivistic presentations of statistics—often with little curricular time dedicated to them—which was one way in which the social sciences were, to paraphrase Gattinella, not accurately reflecting social science. In addition to teaching inaccurate or decontextualized information, the language and framing of "implicit bias" makes it seem like being prejudiced is normal and biological and thus absolves the person doing the implicit bias from wrongdoing, as legal scholar Jonathan Kahn has argued.[4]

In describing one of the downsides of the limited time dedicated to the social sciences, Dr. Engle, a white male clinical faculty member, recalled how they covered "racial associations with poor health care access or demographics of the HIV epidemic as illustrative of some inequities in health" in his school's course. According to Engle, there were "adverse student reactions to it because it feels like profiling." He described how students brought to his attention that it was problematic "if the only times in the curriculum being African American is mentioned is when that person has HIV or they have sickle cell anemia." Showing how connected curricular design and implementation were, Engle argued that many of these problems started at the level of curricular design because they "haven't done a good job across the curriculum" and therefore "early adopters like me doing this stuff can be undermined if it's not systematic across the board." Engle illustrated the perils of decontextualized statistics, which in and of itself can be problematic, as Dr. Carley described in the introduction to this book when she was trying to teach students that uncritically slapping together statistical information could yield horrifyingly racist assumptions about health behaviors and disease prevalence.

While didactic material on race was taught in the lecture setting, clinical faculty members more frequently included information about the salience of race in hypothetical cases that students solved and discussed in the POM small-group setting. With mock cases, students practiced how they would apply the knowledge for clinical use. Jeff, a white male medical student, described a common scenario that medical students were taught in these cases whereby a biological understanding of race was given. He said: "Like, for example, sarcoidosis. If you ever go to anyone who has gone through med school and you say, '[T]hirty-year-old black woman with a cough.' Step 1 will teach you that that is sarcoidosis. Like that is the answer before you even hear anything. But if you said, '[T]hirty-year-old white woman with a cough,' then they'd be like I have no idea; it could be anything."

Jeff's invocation of "step 1" indicates that the United States Medical Licensing Exam (USMLE) would expect a future physician to associate the racial group–symptom pairing of "black woman with a cough" with the disease state of "sarcoidosis," a finding consistent with the fears expressed by social scientists in my study. Another student, Jan, a Black male medical student, said that they "weren't really taught about actual racism but about . . . you know . . . a lot of the diseases that are pre-indicative of race," noting that they were taught biological conceptualizations of race as part of another set of facts he had to memorize, like the racial "correction" for a patient's kidney function. Clinical faculty members and students described curricular content where race was depicted as a biological risk factor or as genetic associations between a racial minority group and a particular disease. This problematic social scientific content was epistemically consistent with the presentation of biomedical or clinical information, as facts about groups of patients. In that sense, it is understandable that, given their lack of social scientific expertise, clinical faculty members would teach these topics in these ways.

These findings about the inaccurate and dangerous depictions of race are consistent with a growing body of scholarship on how racism is built into biomedical and social scientific knowledge.[5] Other case studies of individual school curricular practices have pointed to similar problems, particularly with instruction on race.[6] As sociologist Ruha Benjamin has argued in relationship to cultural conceptualizations of social groups, what she calls "culture talk" acts to obscure "the social reality of those it purports to describe and hides the positionality of those who engage in such descriptions."[7] In addition to clinical faculty members providing students with biological and cultural framings of the salience of race, educators did not regularly include lecture- or case-based didactic material where race was defined as social. Nor did they discuss racism outright.

Jeremy, a white medical student, felt like his school and profession were "not particularly interested" in discussions of race beyond biological or cultural "facts" and that the social constructionist understanding of race could be considered absent. He told me:

We're defining disparities by race, so we have to talk about what race is. The idea of defining race as like "a system of oppression based on perceived differences" is not defined. I think medicine is not particularly interested in that . . . they'll throw out "Black people have this, or Hispanic people have this" . . . essences of race are sort of lumped together and then there's not really a conversation about "well, are these real, scientific distinctions that we're drawing between populations?"

In addition to describing the positivistic presentation of social science in his school's curriculum, Jeremy contrasted the formal didactic material with the nonexistent material. While Jeremy came to medical school with a critical understanding of social categories, this instruction could lead to situations where medical students receive information that goes against what social scientists believe to be a correct representation of the nature, causes, and consequences of social inequalities.

The final way that clinical faculty members engaged in social scientific instruction was by relying on people to share their lived experiences, which also drew on the clinical faculty members' extant repertoire. They witnessed social inequalities in their clinic, and so it was epistemically consistent that they would want to utilize that source of social scientific knowledge in their own instruction. They thought that students sharing information about their background would allow students to imagine how they would react in a clinical setting to a patient that was socially different from them. For example, when I asked Riva, a white student in her third year of medical school, whether she learned any social science, she said she "didn't know," revealing how little was taught (or retained). To follow up, I asked if she was taught anything about gender or race. She explained:

> Students are asked to share about their own culture or racial background and then sort of discuss how that influences their work or how that would inform their work. It's run by physicians and it's not usually always people who have any particular training in like, diversity training or anything like that. So I think sometimes the conversation sort of glides on the experience of the students.

Riva's remarks showed how little her school had done to fulfill LCME Standard 7 if she thought that these faculty members needed training in diversity rather than in the social sciences. But in addition to highlighting the inexperience of faculty members, Riva's remarks pointed to how educators explicitly asked students to share about their social experiences, thus enacting the conscripted curriculum.

Because clinical faculty members lacked the expertise to facilitate these conversations and did not provide students with social scientific data and concepts to work with, and because they decided to teach these courses in a small-group setting rather than in a lecture setting, students did the majority of the work themselves. With these curricular practices, conversations for learning about social sciences depended on students sharing experiences; the pedagogical logic here was that in conscripting students to share these experiences, students would learn about experiences that would be applicable in a clinical setting where there were socially diverse patients. Dismissing these practices as simply rhetorical overlooks the fact that these curricular practices were productive. Even if they were extolling the importance of learning the social sciences, many educators in my sample referred to this space as the "soft" side of medicine, invoking a hard-scientific knowledge versus soft skills divide. These clinical faculty members often established a contrast between clinical "facts" presented in a didactic setting with tested-on material, on the one hand, and social "experience" from the lives of students and patients, on the other. I call the impacts of this established contrast the *anecdotalization effect*.

A by-product of clinical witnessing, the anecdotalization effect happens when clinical faculty members taught the content on social inequalities through examples of lived experience while the bulk of the curriculum focused on systematically gathered knowledge. Thus, one of the biggest results of these curricular practices is the transformation of lessons about social inequalities into anecdotes, reifying an individualizing epistemology that obscures the consideration of structural conditions from view. Other scholars have shown how anecdotes in academic or professional settings are seen as "epistemologically disadvantageous" and, given that status, they are not appreciated, regardless of their veracity.[8] Of course, lived experience can be important for understanding social inequalities, but the focus on experience in the context of the other curricular practices and over-all organization of the medical school created the conditions under which the social sciences were both devalued and constrained. By conscripting students or having patient-led panels about social experiences with health or health care, the clinical faculty members were sending a message, whether they meant it or not, that they did not really care what was taught in these sessions because in all other teaching scenarios, student learning was hypercontrolled—in other words, they were not using social experiences in cardiology lectures. In this sense, conscription was a form of management because the students' telling of their experiences was delimited to this particular time and space, and critical social science was not part of the over-arching curricular picture.

The clinical witnessing perspective centers the physician as the witness rather than as a social being in their own right, and conceptualizes social scientific knowledge on the individual level rather than on the institutional or structural level. As other scholars have documented, clinical faculty members' limited understandings of social inequalities can have a negative impact on patient care. For example, MD-PhD Brooke Cunningham and colleagues have shown how clinicians' uncertainty around the meaning and application of race in clinical encounters can lead to errors in medical decision making, and psychologist Michelle van Ryn and her team have detailed how implicit bias influences clinical decision making to the detriment of racial minorities.[9] In an interview-based study, sociologists Jaime Manzer and Ann Bell have shown that the strategies that clinicians use to minimize or explain away their own bias are oriented around shrouding bias in scientific objectivity and utilizing coded language to describe cultural stereotypes.[10] These understandings, therefore, matter, and with clinical faculty members' enactment of their social scientific curricular practices in the classroom, they ultimately did very little to address the equity problems that the LCME standards purportedly addressed—and that they, themselves, seemed to want to address.

Their lack of social scientific expertise and clinical witnessing perspective combined to provide students with decontextualized, inaccurate, inequitable, and/or anecdotal approaches to understanding social inequalities.

TRANSFORMING THE HUMANITIES INTO INTERPERSONAL TOOLS FOR PLACATION

Clinical faculty members also centered themselves in their approach to incorporating the humanities in the classroom. Many of them engaged in these curricular practices because they thought they were doing the right thing. They thought the humanities would make their lives better, either through catharsis or enrichment; the actual content of the humanities and their disciplinary distinctions did not really matter because what was given to students was diluted or obliquely humanistic content. Clinical faculty members simultaneously trivialized and transformed the value of the humanities. They trivialized the humanities by placing them in electives with nonexperts and transformed them into interpersonal tools of placation, either placating the trainee, the potential patient, or the image of the profession.

Clinical faculty members first transformed the humanities into therapeutic tools for physicians and students. As discussed in chapter 2, educators and students alike spoke about how incredibly stressful the medical education pathway was, begetting the need for something, anything, that would address the empathy problems. Clinical faculty members personally felt the effects of the burnout crisis in their own clinical work and felt that students needed a type of therapeutic support the humanities could offer. Their incorporation of humanities-as-journaling was common in the classroom. Students and faculty members explained the value of writing as inhering in its capacity for expression and release, areas that were perceived as either neglected or in need of "self-care." They emphasized how the individual needed to care for themselves, a point I will return to after describing the content of these humanities electives in more detail.

Dr. Kling, a white male clinical faculty member who oversaw the curricular design for his school's UME, described the purpose of letting students write as "direct[ing] students to behaviors that we hoped would be more fulfilling, meaningful, and less stressful." John, a white male medical student, said, "I think writing helps [some of my peers] kind of cope—like medicine's pretty stressful, it can help them cope, you know—with everything they see." In these humanities electives, clinical faculty members often had students engage in reflection pieces without any structure, analysis, or feedback so that they served as a space for something akin to a diary entry. Students responded to prompts or experiences they had in the classroom or on the wards. These curricular practices were *not* the same as reading and discussing the horrors of medical experimentation or learning "Narrative Medicine" techniques for active interpretation utilized in some critical curricular practices.[11]

Students echoed clinical faculty members' remarks. Andrew, a white male medical student, said that his humanities elective was "a fun thing that people do that's not medicine." Jackie, a white female medical student, said that her book club during her clerkship year was "flexible and it was a nice departure from our everyday clinical activity." She continued, "I can't tell you the last time that I read a book for pleasure because all the other reading material would be science and medicine related because you always have more to learn." The clinical faculty members encouraged therapeutic ends for the humanities. These curricular practices placated the student-clinician self. These students' experiences of these humanities courses as therapeutic were not a coincidence: some educators purposefully taught stress relief or other emotional coping exercises in these humanities offerings. "The Healer's Art"™, described in chapter 3, was very much oriented this way. In fact, in the expressive course description for "The Healer's Art"™, it showed how the course was centered around work on the self: "*your* own humanity . . . *your* sense . . . *your* ability . . . for *ourselves*" (emphasis added). The course also explicitly linked this self-care work with professional burnout, underscoring how clinical experience served as a filter through which clinical faculty members viewed the humanities—both the physician and the self were centered, leaving the patient and also the institutions and systems beyond the curricular frame.

The second transformation of the humanities into an interpersonal tool of placation was far more nefarious. Here, the humanities were weaponized for placating the patient. As scholars of both therapeutic culture and affective capitalism have argued elsewhere, therapeutic discourse can be mobilized as an agent for more calculating professional gains—where employers manipulate therapeutic discourse to maximize the affective control they have over their employees, all with an eye toward increased output and productivity to improve the organization's bottom line.[12] Recent work on the instrumentalization of clinical empathy has revealed how the emotional comportment of clinicians has increasingly become managed by the hospital or profession.[13] Clinical faculty members, knowingly or not, used the humanities as tools for affective control.

Dr. Donovan, a white male humanist and instructor of a literature and medicine elective, elaborated on this instrumentalization by saying: "I think that the whole issue of empathy and compassion . . . there's a real concern that these can be perceived as either patronizing or condescending at best and manipulative at worst. You know I win your trust, and you really like me, then I can get you to agree to an operation that maybe you don't need. But I say, '[O]h I really understand your pain.'" This rationale undergirding what Donovan experienced was further exemplified by the remarks of another white male clinical faculty member, Dr. Stephens, who said that "the relevance and applicability is sometimes viewed rather concretely . . . something that may be important for having a sense of a broader sense of humanity seem less applicable than something that is more clinical and perhaps more immediately useful." The immediate clinical utility that places the physician at the center and the patient as something to be understood was light years away from some of the profession-wide goals regarding the inclusion of the humanities.

Some students picked up on this narrow, instrumentalized vision of the humanities. Gyi, the student who had participated in a "Literature in Medicine" elective, noted its therapeutic orientation. He was even more critical, calling the elective a "glorified communications seminar." He described the literature element being "a little bit neutered because now it is just gone off like a check box on your standardized patient form. Did you shake the patient's hand? Did you drape them appropriately? Did you knock on the door?" When I asked Gyi what he meant by neutered, he explained further: "[L]ike you will not *be* empathetic but we will make it seem like you're the most empathetic person in the room . . . it's about being *perceived* as empathetic." Garrett, a Black male medical student, explained in more detail that the humanities were transformed into tools for ultimately paternalistic and capitalistic gains:

> There are whole studies, like when you sit in a room with a patient on a chair that the perception of time by the patient of how much time you spent in the room nearly doubles. Or, for example, if you make a medical error, and then you say "I'm sorry" to the patient your rate of being sued plummets. There's even a study about the pitch of a surgeon's voice in apologizing to a patient, where surgeons with deeper voices actually get sued more than surgeons with higher ones. There's all this literature and all it boils down to is basically this whole idea of how can you be *seen* like a human, how can you *seem* like a humanist, like fake it til you make it.

Critical here is the notion that *affects* are pivotal to *effects*, whereby "physicians who display a warm, friendly, and reassuring manner are more effective" with their patients.[14] Fake it (e.g., perform humanism) until you make it (e.g., get the clinical outcome you want).

A corollary example can be found in sociologist Alexandra Vinson's study of clinical faculty members teaching communication skills to medical students. Vinson showed the rhetorical power of "patient empowerment" practices, or a set of communication tools that clinical faculty members utilized to convince patients to follow their treatment recommendations by persuading patients to think that it was their idea in the first place.[15] Empathy, patient empowerment, and other affective states are thus interactional "accomplishments" for the medical profession, what sociologist Kelly Underman refers to as part of "affective governance in medical education."[16] The humanities are incorporated to humanize medicine, but in the process, they are medicalized, that is, turned into tools of the medical profession to maintain its control over both its object of work, patients, as well as its workforce, the clinicians.[17]

The third transformation was about placating the image of the profession. Clinical faculty members' clinical experience and their lack of humanities expertise also manifest as elitist, white, triumphalist approaches to incorporating the humanities. Dr. Pultz, who was already introduced in this chapter, elaborated how "we would love to teach history of medicine but the only people who can teach it are semiretired physicians who have nineteenth-century academia-style interests in history. They want to teach great man narratives." What Pultz drew attention to was that, in the absence of a "real historian," the volunteer corps of "semiretired" clinical faculty members would instruct students on whiggish histories in the classroom. This set of curricular practices bore the most resemblance to the historical valuation of the humanities by the medical profession described in chapter 1 because it celebrated a corpus of white European literature and art as well as triumphalist histories of the great men of medicine—all oriented around the notion of the elite, "cultivated" physician. They were the pedagogical instantiations of the hallways of medical schools that display custom portraits of old white men.[18]

Not only did the hallways display old white men, but they also showcased students and faculty members' artwork. Doctors Who

Create, a community of physicians engaged in the humanities, points to similar "giants" as their influences. And of their sixteen listed staff members, fourteen received professional degrees from Ivy League schools; nine also received their undergraduate degrees from Ivy League schools, further speaking to this elite pedigree.[19] For another profession-wide group, the Health Humanities Consortium (HHC), twenty-four of the twenty-five past and present leaders listed on the leadership page were white. In the latest reading list for "compassionate clinicians" put out by the Gold Foundation, which is one of the central philanthropic organizations encouraging more humanistic health care, whiteness is again on display: of the twelve books, ten are by white authors.[20] Similar booklists were given for humanities electives, such as the following course description for a medical school course in my sample: "This course will use close reading of classic literature to explore questions of mortality, ethics, and compassion that arise in the practice of medicine . . . Readings will include fiction and nonfiction by William Carlos Williams, Anton Chekhov, Peter Shaffer, Leo Tolstoy, Mary Shelley, John Updike, and others." In upholding these "canonical" texts, medical schools were upholding a particular race and class as timeless, that of the white elite—and mostly men. William Carlos Williams epitomized venerating not only white elite men but also the profession because he was a clinician and poet.

It was almost as if the types of humanities that were celebrated by the clinical faculty members were frozen in time, as if the conception of these disciplines had not evolved with the disciplines themselves, as if the profession was holding onto an outdated vision of elite status. Perhaps it was also a vestige of paternalistic moral cultivation, like the hubristic belief that it (the medical profession) needed to be the guardian of a particular vision of *who* a doctor could be—that members of the profession were not just number-crunching biomedical robots but cultured, cultivated, well-rounded people. The decisions that these clinical faculty members made to engage in triumphalist or therapeutic transformations of the humanities in their electives must also be construed as actively hostile because they were leaving out the important critical scholarship from humanities fields that call out the inhumanities that the medical profession has propagated.

* * *

While many of the problems that accompany the delivery of social sciences and humanities material starts with the curricular design, the interpretive work of the clinical faculty members who enact the curricular practices in the classroom present additional problems. Clinical faculty members decontextualized and devalued the social sciences while transforming the humanities for triumphalist and therapeutic purposes. It was a striking juxtaposition to see where data—these "studies" showing how performing empathy yields better patient satisfaction ratings—were invoked in the instruction of medical students. They were given that data but not data on the history of medical experimentation. Taken together, in delivering the problematic content in the classroom, clinical faculty members reached for lessons that assumed, reinforced, and glorified a conflation of professional clinician with the white elite. What the clinical faculty members decided to include for classroom instruction was just as important as what they decided to leave out. What was obscured was a constructivist, structural, and systemic understanding of how social categories could shape their future patients' lives and own clinical practices. To round out my portrait of this process of knowledge application, I will turn my attention in chapter 5 to what students take away from these curricular practices and the other lessons that clinical faculty members impart.

5

RECEIVING
CURRICULAR PRACTICES

When I asked a white female medical student, Caroline, if she had learned anything from the social sciences in her medical school so far, she said that she didn't know. As I went through several follow-up questions to see what, if anything, she learned about the relationship between race and health— or gender and health—she still did not have anything to share. I then asked her if she had heard of the term "cultural competence," which was one of the explicit Liaison Committee on Medical Education (LCME) standards (Standard 7.6). She said yes, so I followed up by asking her what she thought "culture" meant. She told me, "[W]e don't get tested on the information we receive so I can't give you a definition of culture." Caroline went on to explain that the part of the overall curriculum at her medical school where they learned about LCME Standard 7 was quite brief. She explained that all 170 students in her cohort were "required to attend lectures and panel presentations that covered ethics, cultural competency, professionalism, and medical malpractice" in one single week.

One week and that was it.

Caroline said that the panel presentations were often given by members of the LGBTQ community or people with disabilities. Similar to the way that case-based or conscripted curricular practices deliver social scientific information as anecdotes, panel presentations relied on people with lived experience and with specific social identities or illnesses to share their experiences with the medical students and faculty members. At this point in the interview, Caroline and I had developed a good enough rapport and she was laughing at how little she recalled from these sessions. I felt comfortable asking her that if she could not remember how to define culture, then was there anything else that stood out to her from the week? She had two examples. The first was that her class was given a map of the city their medical school was in with the life expectancies in U.S. Census tracks; the second was that they were shown a video on Chinese cupping and traditional healing that covered how to recognize when these practices were dangerous for patient health. I concluded this part of the interview by asking Caroline what she thought the goal of the course was. She said, "[A]n opportunity to look at the non-science parts, but a lot of that is not applicable until the third or fourth year."

This conversation with Caroline illustrates how curricular designers and implementers impart lessons to students. For the social scientific lessons, Caroline detailed the curricular structure and thus showed how clinical faculty members at her school chose to shoehorn social sciences into an already stocked curriculum, giving social sciences only a single week of instruction time. As Dr. Li, an Asian male clinical faculty member, noted in our interview, his school's approach to instructing the social sciences left students "feeling like, well, if something's twelve weeks, then it must be more important than something that is one week. We don't intend to send this message but that's exactly what ends up happening." Like Li, clinical faculty members aimed to incorporate social sciences into undergraduate medical education (UME) to address educational requirements that were established to help make health care more equitable. In practice, however, their approach perpetuated social inequalities. For example, by describing the panel presentations and lecture content, Caroline pointed to her clinical faculty members' inaccurate and inequitable interpretation of the social sciences: culture was exoticized (e.g., Chinese cupping), mortality statistics were given without context (e.g., life expectancies by U.S. Census tract), and anecdotal experiences were prioritized (e.g., LGBTQ patient panel), and these lessons were not incentivized (e.g., no exam). Finally, Caroline's invocation at the end, where she said that the social scientific content was not applicable until her third or fourth year—when she would rotate through clinical clerkships—pointed to her understanding that it was through clinical experience that she would appreciate the value of these topics.

Students described similar experiences with the humanities content. When I asked Scott, a Black male medical student, about the humanities courses at his medical school, he described his school's adoption of "The Healer's Art"™. He thus highlighted how central clinical experience—and experience more broadly—was to the value of the humanities:

> We had one course that was started . . . I forget her name, but she's pretty much had her whole career at UCSF [University of California, San Francisco] and just kind of made her career out of . . . the human component of healing. So it was all about addressing emotion, your own emotion, the patient's emotion, the family's emotion, the social dynamic emotions and recognizing that and how one of the most important things to being a good physician or just provider in general is bringing your human component into it. So it's like you all are twenty-five years or older, you have twenty-five years of experience dealing with humans and that's the most important part.

After drawing attention to the prestigious medical school and the entire career made "out of the human component of healing" background of "The Healer's Art"™ creator, Scott showed how the course was oriented around tapping into experience rather than lessons from the humanities disciplines themselves. Students learned that they have this experience being human and that is all they would need to tap into. This was the simultaneous trivializing and transforming of the humanities that I outlined in chapter 4, but what I want to note here is how this curricular approach reinforced the primacy of experience as *the* source of knowledge.

In addition to learning lessons about clinical experience as paramount, many students did not really see the point of what the clinical faculty members were trying to teach them. Instead of viewing these curricular experiences as "a waste of time," as many students put it, I draw attention in this chapter to the subtle socialization that occurred via these productive and ideological curricular practices. The clinical faculty members, through their decisions regarding curricular design and implementation, relayed significant lessons to students about what knowledge was valuable, who was an expert, and how to be a professional in ways that reproduced social inequalities and the status quo. I highlight specifically how these lessons converged to create an ideological socialization that continued to reinforce that the image of the professional physician was one who was white and elite, did not need to understand social inequalities, and fell in line.

I present a few lessons that students reported they learned that went beyond—or built on some of—the explicit lessons detailed in prior chapters. First, I detail how students depict both the social sciences and the humanities as a "waste of time" relative to the importance of the rest of their curriculum. I focus on how they learn to value biomedical knowledge and faculty-members-as-instructors compared to devaluing social scientific and humanistic knowledge and students-as-instructors. Then I describe how students from marginalized backgrounds were more likely to be placed in positions as instructors for content that was devalued as a "waste of time" or distinctly "not medicine." They found this devolution of responsibility as both unfair and burdensome. Next, I focus on students who resisted and attempted to change curricular practices at their schools, particularly with the social sciences, and show how those students largely met apathy or repression from their schools' leaders. I end the chapter showing how this apathy or repression happened alongside lessons that students learned from the humanities content—lessons that encouraged docility and stoked status anxiety.

THE MEANING OF MEANINGLESSNESS

Compared to clinical faculty members, students often had very different impressions of the efficacy of and implications for how the social sciences were taught. I felt such a palpable gap between students' skepticism and educators' enthusiasm. Clinical faculty members' curricular practices, to my knowledge, were not *intentionally* marginalizing. Nonetheless, their decisions around how to incorporate the social sciences and humanities into their school's curricular practices had the effect of rendering the content seemingly meaningless because of where the courses were placed, how they were incentivized, and who was involved with facilitating the learning. But this meaninglessness was meaningful. While a mundane point, it is important nonetheless to remember that curricular practices are productive even when marked by an absence; incorporations of the social sciences and humanities were always considered in comparison to the rest of the biomedical material.

Students such as Dylan, a white male medical student, pointed to how little the social sciences meant at his school:

Yeah, there is an issue there; there is an issue. It comes up, people talk about it, and there are lectures and parts of the curriculum where they intend to address certain issues. They tend to be almost like superfluous kind of lectures where *no one really cares*. Because it's just now we're going to *take a little break* and talk about, you know, the Mediterranean Diet or alternative medicine, how acupuncture and Tai Chi have been known to do this and that. We talked about domestic violence. In general, maybe it was just our institution, but these topics were not very well addressed [emphasis added].

I asked Dylan what he thought his educators' objectives were for teaching this content. He retorted: "[T]o broaden the narrow-mindedness of medical students." When I then asked whether that was explicitly conveyed or his impression, he explained: "[B]ecause I've heard the course director talk about it, because we are [narrow minded]. We're trained to be that way." Dylan continued explaining how "we spend four years learning very narrowly, like one side of your brain, one very specific type of information, one specific type of learning. Ultimately it's such a time crunch that you don't get to explore other things." Looping back to the course, Dylan concluded, "[A]gain, it was a dedicated hour every week where we could talk about something that wasn't science. It *could have been anything*; we could have talked about painting [emphasis added]."

As interview after interview revealed, the sentiments that "no one really cares" and that the presentation of social sciences and humanities content were "a little break" did not happen only at Dylan's institution. Most student respondents said that their medical school did not signal that understanding how social inequalities affect their patients' or peers' lives was an important area to master. Many students *laughed*—more often than not, sarcastically; other times, awkwardly—when I asked if they were taught about racism's effects on patients because they were certain that they had not been taught anything of the sort.

Students noted that faculty-presented information was what medical students *really* needed to know. Chris, a white male medical student, said that social scientific instruction on racism was "just not what we are there for . . . we spend two years learning basic science and when you spend most of your day learning about pharmacology and pathology and physiology that all of a sudden 'the social' seems less relevant . . . it's not on the test that's coming up. It's a life skill but it's not a medical school skill, one you have to learn to get an A on the test." Anna, a white female medical student, mirrored Chris's remarks, stating, "[I]t's hard because your time is limited, because at the end of the day it doesn't matter if you understand how race is important for medicine or if you were involved with the urban underserved . . . you still have to get good grades, you have all these tests you have to do well on." White medical students in particular felt that the instruction of social scientific content did not really matter; they did not feel that they, as white people, were implicated because the format and delivery made it seem like race was a nonwhite person's experience or problem. They did not have to care. This finding was particularly important regarding the future of the medical profession and who students believed has a responsibility to serve marginalized populations.[1]

The language choices that Chris and Anna used underscore how these lessons were oriented around perceptions of clinical relevance for medical education. Understanding racism was a "life skill" but "not a medical school skill" because at "the end of the day it doesn't matter" whether students know structural social scientific knowledge. Gyi, a South Asian male medical student, also invoked this bottom line for medical education when I spoke to him about his curricular experiences with social sciences. He summarized the lessons imparted to him by saying, "I think in reality, at the *end of the day* like yeah, it's great if you learn about, you know, the proper way to use pronouns with LGBT patients. But like, you know if you fail your cardiology exam, you have to repeat the year, you know what I mean?" Gyi showed starkly what messaging they received about the relative unimportance of social science data as well as about the heteronormativity that was embedded in medical education.[2]

The humanities were also understood by students to lack relevance, which was far afield from the clinical faculty members' curricular dreams. Darren, a white male medical student who had taken an art elective, put it bluntly, "[R]elevance to a student is whether questions make it on the test or not . . . the humanities stuff that we were learning about almost sounds like a waste of time because we want to pass the tests. I have to stress to you just how bullshit these classes are." The weight placed on the humanities in the overall curricular structure was pertinent for influencing how seriously the majority of students approached the subject; but so was the epistemic value. The flexibility of this elective structure did not encourage structural change—but then again, neither did the content of these courses. Dr. Donovan, a white male humanist, said that he quickly learned that he could not expect medical students to read because they "are usually trained in the culture where they don't do extensive reading." Dr. Sampson, a white female humanist, backed up Donovan by saying: "You can't organize your classroom thinking 'well great, so everyone will have read this so that will be our platform, and we'll launch from there.' Nope you can't do that; what you have to do is find like the key three paragraphs and then okay let's read these together. Because it's not that they won't read, but they'll only read things that they think are really vital and a poem that is not going to be it yet." Just like with the social sciences, active and thoughtful engagement with the humanities was not conveyed as valuable by the profession.

Again, it was distinctly in relation to biomedical knowledge and the "rest" of medical school that the humanities were constructed as a fun break. Jeremy, a white male medical student, explained how the value of biomedical knowledge was reinforced by who they were taught were valuable in their profession: "[Y]our goal is to become a bigwig in a biomedical research lab." Lindsay, a multiracial female medical student, described the value of biomedical knowledge as being signaled by the content and magnitude of knowledge they were expected to know: "[L]ike here are 5,000 flashcards on bio facts, please remember all of them by Friday."[3] Clinical and biomedical knowledge were the most important. The curricular practices were set up to cater to those with biomedical backgrounds, but it was done in a way that also reinforced the social status quo. For example, Lindsay explained how the clinical faculty member in charge of curricular development at her medical school said that they could not require a course on the social sciences because students have different levels of exposure to the social sciences. She said they told her that: "[T]here's just no way to bridge that gap . . . you have people who have a degree in sociology and some people have never heard about it before, so you can't just teach a standard class." But as Lindsay insightfully noted, "[T]hat is just not true because clearly they have expectations for other disciplines . . . the first day of biochemistry I sat next to somebody who had a PhD in biochem and I had never taken a biochem course in my life."

Interestingly, the students parroted what clinical faculty members said about their basic sciences peers stymying real reform. They described the biomedical people as the ones who needed the humanities and social sciences content the most but also as the ones who would not pursue it. For example, Flannery, a white female medical student, told me: "I hear young students say all the time like 'oh, I hate this small group, oh, I hate culture and diversity credits, oh, I hate the humanities requirements.' It's also just some of them are science people; they're just not humanities people, you know?" Flannery described a "science" person as one who was not interested in "culture and diversity," thus revealing her understanding of a prototypical "science" person.

As Caroline explained, "[T]he people that need it the most are not the people who are benefitting from the humanities content because they are not taking it seriously or they want to do research instead . . . the gunners aren't doing some of the humanities stuff." "Gunners" are medical students who were perceived to be incessantly competitive, always gunning to attain the best in class, best residency program, best fellowship, and then best clinical faculty positions. The "gunners" were portrayed as more likely than others to be more concerned with learning biomedical knowledge and thus more likely to conceptualize the humanities content as a "waste of time."[4] In these scenarios, where the bigwig biomedical gunners were devaluing this content, they were also describing this content as a drag, as optional, or as "entirely debatable"—to use Jeremy's words—as opposed to the essential biomedical information.

TAXING THE ALREADY MARGINALIZED

Another core lesson that students received was through the clinical faculty members' communication about *who* possessed valued expertise. In the practice of medicine (POM) small groups, clinical faculty members conscripted their students into social sciences instruction. But they were setting up these students for devaluation because this practice was premised on the presence of people whose social identities conferred a form of experientially based expertise, which contrasted with the presentation of factual knowledge throughout the rest of the curriculum that was uniformly provided by faculty. Not only did "no one really care" about the social sciences or humanities, but they also learned not to care about those doing that pedagogical labor. Robyn, a white female medical student, recounted a memory of when it felt like the medical school did not even *consider* Black students as learners. As she recalled, "[W]e have one small-group scenario on like a Black patient who wants to see a Black doctor, which I think is a great exercise for the white students to think about 'how do I do this,' but not particularly inclusive of Black students who are like 'this assignment is not written with me in mind as a student, like you were discounting my presence here.'" The curricular practices were set up for white students and the decisions that clinical faculty members made had distinct and disparate effects on marginalized students relative to their privileged peers.

Clinical faculty members' reliance on student participation to discuss social inequalities did not—in and of itself—have to reproduce social inequalities. As I described in chapter 3, however, within the same explanation of the benefits that the small group bestowed upon students regarding the instruction of social inequalities, clinical faculty members often pointed to the *demographic* composition of their student body within these small groups. I found that clinical faculty members were therefore more likely to conscript students of color in the instruction of race, or queer students in the instruction of sexuality—and that these students felt (understandably) unfairly burdened by this work.

The numerical rarity of marginalized students in medical school often meant that they were the *only* student of their underrepresented background to share their experiences. This could be isolating, as Mark, a white male medical student, pointed out. He noted how his friends of color were upset that they had to carry this burden because his "school is not like—well med school in general is very homogenous—there is not a lot of diversity." He continued, saying: "I've been lucky to be around people who have taught me about it . . . I think race comes up a lot more when people of color are in those small groups and then bring up the fact that this has been my experience, da-da-da. They basically have to be the catalyst for it to even be on the table." As a result of having to be conscripted in this way more often, marginalized students described experiences that added to their workload and emotional burden.

This finding was made abundantly clear by the students of color that I interviewed. As Marian, a Black female medical student, said, "I spent a lot of time in my first year trying to educate people, students and faculty alike . . . I'm constantly the only Black person in this small group because there are five of us in the whole school." As we talked, it became clear that what was most bothersome to her was not only what she had to do but also how it made her feel. She told me, "[I]t has been a lot. I spent a lot of time in my first year trying to educate people, students and faculty alike, and it's so exhausting to have to do that . . . it's so exhausting I feel like, it's not my role to educate you—you can use Google." As Marian's account suggested, teaching her peers and faculty members was not her job, and the exhaustion stemmed from feeling like she had to engage in this type of instruction. Her comment that students and faculty members could "use Google" pointed to her frustration in having to bear the instructor's burden in her small group.

To drive the point home, Lindsay, a multiracial female student, articulated the broader significance of why student-led sessions were perceived as less important: the medical school "would never ask students to teach anatomy even if there was a change that needed to be made. Even if they were really great students, they would *hire somebody* whose job it is to examine and teach that." Anatomy, deemed important, was taught by faculty, whereas critical social sciences were considered "not essential for every physician." Because clinical faculty members decided to teach social sciences by relying on experience, where structural knowledge was sacrificed at the altar of the individual, it placed students who were socially "different"—that is, not white, not upper class, not cisgender, not heterosexual—in a position to teach their peers. Thus, students who were not facsimiles of the current professional leadership were unfairly taxed and had more work than their peers, and reported more emotional exhaustion as a result. In a curricular context in which the social scientific material was devalued relative to other curricula, these students did work that was rendered futile or meaningless, furthering their disillusionment.

STUDENT RESISTANCE

The curricular injustice detailed so far led many students to take their concerns to the clinical faculty members to reform the way that race in particular was taught. Students of color described mixed receptions from clinical faculty when they addressed their concerns. While some students of color were met with reprimand, other students of color encountered different types of "opportunities" for change. The students of color painted a not-so-rosy narrative of how much of an "opportunity" they were really being given by their clinical faculty superiors, often describing how they were given a platform to bring matters to their superiors, but it was often an empty platform without any actual opportunities for tangible change.

For example, Scott, a Black male medical student, recounted what he felt he was up against: "So the very first lecture of first year it was all 'race is biological' and even some talk of 'one drop theory.' At the end of that lecture, I sent a very strongly worded email to the professor and brought it up with the dean. I was real disappointed when the next year the same thing happened." While Scott had the "opportunity" to voice his concerns and had many discussions as part of this opportunity, the curriculum remained unchanged. While I cannot know why it did not change, the disorganization of the medical school certainly could not have helped. Speaking to this disorganization as a student at a different school was Lindsay, who felt that she was actually quite "lucky":

> Frankly in medical school, students are so transient. You come in, you don't really know what's going on, by the time you do, you only have a year left. It's both really, really lovely and also simultaneously disheartening to see that every year students come in with the same calls, with the same critiques, with the same efforts and writing and proposals and meetings literally year by year by year and we share them and they're identical . . . I think beyond that is I suppose we're really lucky that the biggest opposition that we face is apathy or lack of urgency whereas talking to medical students and people from other schools, they're more . . . explicitly shut down or discouraged.

As Lindsay noted, she was "lucky" in the sense that she was not "explicitly shut down or discouraged," but these organizational roads to nowhere yielded no change. Thus, the disorganized structure seemed to absorb the students' curricular critiques.

For the students of color in my study, the opportunities to resist their school's curricular failures were inseparable from the costs. Students confronted indifference from administration, faculty members, and other students regarding their requests to include content on structural inequalities, remove content containing problematic presentations about social inequalities, and be protected from the exhausting need to explain their experiences to their faculty members and peers. These episodes were akin to what other scholars called "identity taxation" or "racialized equity labor," where people in marginalized positions are expected to do labor (often unpaid or undercompensated) as a result of their social identity.[5] These moments of marginalization were all connected. In many schools, if students of color did not do this labor of instructing their peers and faculty members about race and racism, then all students lacked the actual curricular content (because clinical faculty members thought that the instruction should emanate from those with lived experience). Students of color then *became* the curricular content when clinical faculty members enacted the conscripted curriculum in the POM small groups. Even worse, however, was that the intellectual and emotional labor of students of color was not valued.

For example, Lisa, a Black female medical student, explained a situation to me when she got in trouble for raising concerns about the way they were talking about race in the POM small group. As she recounted, "I got some shit from one of my facilitators . . . they're like 'oh, well, your activism is getting in the way of your studies.'" Lisa's frustration and disillusionment were unmistakable. She continued as if she were talking to these clinical faculty members who were giving her a hard time: "Well maybe you mother fuckers should like do something about what I'm saying, then I wouldn't have to do anything. I could just pay attention." Students who pushed back on how their clinical faculty members decided to teach race confronted what Angelique Davis and Rose Ernst have called *racial gaslighting*, or "the political, social, economic, and cultural processes that perpetuate and normalize a white supremacist reality though pathologizing those who resist."[6] In studies of the medical profession, scholars have noted how physicians are unwilling to be whistleblowers and are strongly encouraged to handle problems "in house" as part of protecting their professional autonomy relative to other stakeholders (e.g., hospital administrators).[7] Jonathan, a Latino medical student, imitated himself in response to this type of socialization: "I'm always like 'oh you told me to do it? I'll go do it. I'm a good little soldier.'"

Lisa's story showed that the impact on student learning and marginalized students had a feedback loop, doubly burdening them. Lisa was doing the work to participate in conversations about race—as she was asked to do. Yet when she did so in a way that could force more critical attention to the topic, her efforts were brushed aside as "activism" and depicted as interfering with her *real* studies, further reinforcing the ideological values of the medical profession.[8] Her final exasperated remarks about how she "wouldn't have to do anything," she could "just pay attention," if the faculty members just did their jobs and taught the social sciences was telling of the broader situation in which the clinical faculty members had not assumed responsibility for this instruction. Student activism—and students' accounts of how medical schools react to activism with dismissal, false empowerment, devolution unto students, and reprimand—demonstrated many medical school leaders' stubborn commitment to retaining the status quo. At the same time that clinical faculty members engaged in these pro-biomedical and pro-white lessons, they also engaged in humanities-based curricular practices that were oriented toward socializing students to be docile.

REPRODUCING THE STATUS QUO

Students received messages about the meaninglessness of the social sciences and humanities, that social inequalities were just a marginalized person's problem, and that resisting the current curricular practices would be futile or potentially career-threatening. They also received lessons about falling in line with the extant professional status quo. Jeremy explained this culture by saying, "[T]he way the information is presented, it's all very authoritarian. You're expected to basically just accept whatever it is that we're given. Spoon-fed information, and for some of it, just repeating after the instructor. There is nothing to really argue with." One way that the clinical faculty members reinforced the status quo was by subtly socializing students to avoid critical thinking, put their heads down, and stick with the biomedical program. These types of messages were also conveyed through the humanities lessons themselves—both in their therapeutic form and triumphalist elevation of Eurocentric art forms.

Caroline, the medical student who opened the chapter, expressed to me that she had wanted to attend humanities offerings at her medical school but had not yet done so. Because of her school's curricular structure, the responsibility to engage with the humanities fell to the students:

> Sometimes I won't make it a priority, and then I'll hear my friend talking about it; yeah, of course, that's what I want to do, like why wouldn't I go to that? Because you just kind of get caught up in like the wrappings of like just getting another test done, you know. But I think those people, and that's what I admire most about them, is that they make it a priority to have different experiences, and to put those experiences first before studying. That can be really hard to do that and also get good grades, you know? But I think it's an individual choice; like all the burden is on you as a student to decide to do that.

While Caroline admired her peers that seemed to have the capacity to engage in the humanities, she also called out her school for devolving the responsibility for taking these courses onto students. Rachel, an Asian female medical student, also felt that the humanities were "yet another thing we have to do on our own." She mentioned that the elective structure and content did nothing to address how medical school was "such a loaded experience and half of it is very isolative, where you just literally teach yourself everything." These students pointed to the irony that these humanities electives, despite being designed to relieve stress, actually put an additional burden on students to take care of their own wellness.

Rather than addressing the original sources of students' depression, exhaustion, and disengagement, clinical faculty members gave students opportunities with the humanities that were originally intended to be cathartic experiences that built up students' resilience and taught them tools for coping. It was precisely because these clinical faculty members did not view the humanities as a challenge to the biomedical status quo, however, that the humanities were incorporated; these clinical faculty members pitched the humanities as a therapeutic, extracurricular support to the *real* curriculum. These curricular practices exposed the way in which medical school was structured to reproduce the status quo (e.g., students teach themselves, there is too much to learn and master, the sources of stress remain unchallenged) and the way organizational flexibility was marshaled to enact this. For the latter point, the structure of integration (e.g., optional, elective, extracurricular) and the valuation of the humanities (e.g., placating the physician, patient, and profession) created the conditions in which the responsibility for alleviating burnout fell squarely with the individual student or physician rather than with the profession or the workplace.

These practices thus create the conditions under which the individual student is charged with handling their own well-being as a way for the profession to address burnout. Being a "good" physician is also being a "good" worker, one who shows "respect for authority, punctuality, cleanliness, docility, and conformity."[9] The status quo, or the existing structure of medical education and corresponding curricular practices, remains protected and unchallenged while the humanities are prescribed by clinical faculty members as patches of placation. The way in which the humanities were medicalized to expand or maintain the profession's jurisdiction and social control over problems meant that they served as a discipline of docility, or a set of tools aimed at rendering medical students agreeable, passive, and focused on themselves.[10] They served a socializing function, transmitting particular lessons about how and when humanizing lessons matter.[11] In this sense, the humanities were tools utilized to coddle the science, technology, engineering, mathematics and medicine (STEMM) disciplines.

In addition to these lessons in docility, another way in which the clinical faculty members chose to include the humanities in UME— with their choice to admit students who were talented in white, Eurocentric, elite art forms—also reproduced the status quo in the medical profession. Perhaps the *inclusion-as-admissions* approach for incorporating the humanities seemed harmless. Why not admit talented superstars? Why not teach literature or history in students' free time? These approaches implied that the parading of humanities content was part of an identity project—it was a luxury to have these (white, elite) students, these courses, this time. The archetype of the medical student who was also a concert pianist—or a poet or impressionist painter—combined the status cues of the old and new elite.[12] The contents of this well-rounded achiever's curriculum vitae harkened back to the *old elite*. With the old elite, from sociologist Shamus Khan's formulation, white Eurocentric forms of culture were celebrated and denoted as marks of distinction—like the so-called canonical fine arts and literature, which was evident in the educators' discussion of students, elective offerings, and syllabi.

But the performance of this privilege also signaled a certain degree of effortlessness, as if these medical students did these activities with ease and as leisure. An ability to do it all is a way to prove worth, which is another, more recent cultural association with leisure and class, best exemplified in Khan's work on the ease and effortlessness of modern class privilege, in what he calls the comportment of the *new elite*. When students "bounce in" and casually remark, "Oh, me? I'm just an incredible scientist *and* concert pianist," they were adopting this interactional style of the new elite. The remark by Jennifer, a Latina medical student, in chapter 3 about her peers was exemplative here. She described a talent show put on by her medical school to showcase "the talent." In mimicking some of the participants, she said, "'[H]ey, you know I had been playing piano since I was two,' or 'I'm a professional this and professional that.'" The casual nature of the "conservatory level" piano playing was essential; it had the effect of making this professional musicianship seem effortless despite clearly having been a life-long endeavor. Attached to the profile of the student who was skilled in the fine arts was also the impression that this student was poised to enjoy and contribute to these bodies of work effortlessly.

Such an effortless profile is consistent with other scholars' work on the oral culture of medical students that construct the idealized physician as cool, calm, and in on the joke.[13] And, there was a running joke among medical students that the Patagonia fleece was a subtle "flex" they all looked forward to—they would appear humble and cozy but would have an expensive jacket showing that they had truly made it. More than the white coat, perhaps, the Patagonia fleece with the school's insignia on the lapel conferred the status of having matriculated into a top residency program. Patagonia fleeces are well made and warm, I am sure, but so are a host of other jacket brands. Patagonia fleeces thus do more than just confer status within medicine—they are the jacket that marks an effortless membership in the upper class. They are the uniform of the new elite.[14] The humanities are like the Patagonia fleeces in how they confer status within medicine because ease is an interactional style that displays comfort, confidence, and self-assuredness—new elite status is what you *do*, not just what you have.[15] The performance of leisure, just like the performance of effortlessness, revealed the culture of medicine but also reinforced its white and elite social identity.

* * *

Although the social sciences and humanities were implemented separately, their impacts on socialization must be viewed collectively.

As the great white men were being upheld as triumphant reminders of the profession's past accomplishments, discussion of the systematic and enduring racism of the medical profession was excluded. Preferred pronouns were taught by a panel of queer patients, but there was no accountability for students to use them, and students learned that they must cope obediently with the horrors of clinical practice by journaling. Medical students were being socialized into an ideological perspective that rewarded docility and prioritized biomedicine. They were being socialized into a profession that reproduced inequalities while maintaining the white elite status quo. When the humanities were seen as a mark of distinction—one that signaled the ease with which such extraordinary achievement was possible—this ease must be compared to the outright struggle most medical students faced. Not only did most students struggle with the slog, misery, and anxiety that this educational phase seemed to elicit, but the students in marginalized social positions were also taxed based on their identities, especially when fighting social injustice. These curricular practices were productive, ideological, and ultimately bent toward injustice.

CONCLUSION

The questions about what physicians need to know to provide humane and equitable care are as old as the profession itself, whether one gestures to the early days of Western allopathic medicine with the Hippocratic Oath or one starts the history of the U.S. medical profession with the consolidation of standards, schools, and authority in the mid-twentieth century. As the U.S. medical profession—and the society in which it is embedded—evolve and become more complex, these debates over what knowledge is needed and how it should be applied have continued apace. Thus, examining debates about curricular practices reveal the medical profession's aspirations for the future, as well as how its members understand their present. The degree to which social sciences and humanities figure into these debates has waxed and waned—and the degree to which the medical profession is reflexive about its relationship with engaging in dehumanizing and inequitable health care has also vacillated. The U.S. medical profession has not done nearly enough, however, to account for its complicity in racist, sexist, capitalist, and cis- and heteronormative systems that perpetuate inequalities and inhumanities.

In this book, I have outlined the process by which the promise of the humanities and social sciences failed to be fully realized in U.S. medical education. These were not merely unrealized dreams; the resulting curricular practices also reproduced and maintained social inequalities. This process of knowledge application, whereby medical educators took the humanities and social sciences and articulated curricular dreams, designed curricular practices, and then implemented them in the classroom, was ultimately a process of compounded failure. Clinical faculty members figured heavily in this process because they were the dreamers, the designers, the implementers; their interpretations of the value of the humanities and social sciences for the clinic patterned how, what, when, where, and why medical students learned material from these fields.

COMPOUNDED FAILURE

At the profession-wide curricular dreaming phase, clinical faculty members—comprising advisory committees of the Liaison Committee on Medical Education (LCME), publishing reports and articles, deliberating at Association of American Medical Colleges (AAMC) meetings—began the knowledge application process. Other educators had a seat at the table at this phase, but clinical faculty members ended up being the most dominant curricular dreamers. They set this process of knowledge application in motion by beginning to conceptualize the need for the humanities and social sciences, filtered through their limited understandings of the problems themselves. Clinical practice, after all, is interpretive work, and that extends to how these needs are understood.[1] In their clinical work, clinical faculty members witnessed or experienced what I have described as two big bodies of problems: *equity problems* and *empathy problems*.

Clinical faculty members witnessed equity problems in their clinical practice. They saw the impacts of social inequalities on the health of their patients; they saw the limits of their biomedical knowledge against the stubborn effects of inequities by class, race, gender, and sexuality. They saw these problems in their clinic, patient after patient, rendering the mode by which clinical faculty members appreciated the equity problems as a mode of other individuals' experiences. This *clinical witnessing* mode of recognizing equity problems was markedly different than, say, reading histories about racism in medicine or learning about structural heteropatriarchy's impacts on health. Clinical faculty members also experienced empathy problems in their clinical practice. They felt the squeeze of a demanding health-care administrative structure that reduced their time with patients. They felt the brutality of observing human suffering. They felt for their fellow physician colleagues, intermittently breaking down amid the various pressures to perform. As with the equity problems, they experienced these problems in their clinical setting; unlike the equity problems, the clinicians were centered as the source of information.

Clinical faculty members felt these empathy problems acutely, yet most of them only witnessed the equity problems because most clinical faculty members at medical schools come from socially privileged backgrounds. The mostly white clinical faculty members in my study seemed to construct the stakes of empathy problems as higher than those of equity problems. With their framing, the burned-out physician was formulated as a source of potential *patient* harm—a consequential leap that the clinical faculty members did not make when discussing the equity problem. In other words, most clinical faculty members did not construct the inequitable physician as dangerously as a burned-out one, despite there being evidence indicating otherwise (even in their own academic journals).[2]

At the curricular dreaming phase, these equity and empathy problems loomed large. Profession-wide curricular initiatives, programming, and standards were aimed at addressing these problems that the clinical faculty members confronted. The LCME standards encapsulated the profession's incorporation of the social sciences for undergraduate medical education (UME); professional initiatives, such as the AAMC's Fundamental Role of the Arts and Humanities for Medical Education (FRAHME), captured how the profession suggested how the humanities should be included. The social sciences were required; the humanities were not. These two bodies of knowledge held inordinate promise at this curricular dreaming phase; much of this clinical faculty member–driven curricular dreaming never moved beyond the vague potential of these fields to solve equity and empathy problems. But clinical faculty members also had more concrete aims, as did the humanities and social sciences scholars working in medical education—at the dreaming phase, curricular solutions abounded.

When articulating concrete aims, still only at the discursive level, medical educators emphasized that future physicians should be able to contextualize health experiences and health inequalities, cultivate critical understandings of the medical profession and knowledge, enhance clinical skills of observation, and augment their reflective capacities. In their view, drawing from the humanities and social sciences would allow clinical faculty members to understand the complexity of human life and the broader structure of inequalities that pattern the lives of patients and providers. At this curricular dreaming phase, the discussions at the profession-wide level were more expansive than what most schools ultimately implemented because each step along the knowledge application pipeline created more opportunity for clinical faculty members to (mis)interpret what the social sciences and humanities could do for physicians. Big ideas fall hard.

Medical schools were set up with a fair amount of *organizational flexibility*. I use the term "flexibility" here because, while it appeared to the observer (me) and inhabitants alike that medical schools were disorganized and chaotic, this was a result of decisions that medical school leaders made. Not only did the organizational flexibility afford each individual medical school's educators the opportunity to interpret the profession-wide guidelines and programming to their own liking, it also placed clinical faculty members in positions of curricular power. Designing or enacting curricular practices in addition to engaging in their clinical and research work, clinical faculty members often rotated through these curricular-centric positions on a semiregular basis, making it unclear who was in charge of what and when. It was a sheer organizational feat at each medical school to have "the 30,000-foot view," as Dr. Brown, a white male humanist, put it.

With clinical faculty members in charge of curricular design, their interpretations were center stage. Their lack of substantive expertise—yet vast clinical experience that they utilized as a proxy for this substantive expertise—came into play. Organizational sociologists have shown that the greater the specificity and clarity of an advocated reform—and the attendant ramifications of failing to comply—the greater the likelihood that the reform will be effective.[3] Clinical faculty members' lack of substantive expertise was an issue precisely because the required social sciences in the LCME standards and suggested humanities programing were not specific or clear.

In moving from curricular dreams to curricular design with the social scientific material, the prism of clinical witnessing—that is, the physicians' appreciation of social inequalities based on their witnessing of inequalities that their patients faced without the structural knowledge that undergirded them—hovered over the knowledge application process. Despite the recognition of the relevance of understanding social inequalities that clinical witnessing conferred, it also constrained the design and enactment of curricular practices. Clinical faculty members made curricular decisions that signaled their limited understanding of social science. In the curricular maps that clinical faculty members created, the social sciences were often shoehorned into insignificant places within the curriculum or relegated into a "Practice of Medicine" (POM) course. When placed in the POM course, clinical faculty members conscripted students from marginalized social positions to share their personal experiences so their (implicitly and sometimes explicitly) white cishet peers and faculty could learn about "the social."

This failure of social scientific knowledge application became compounded once clinical faculty members got to the classroom itself. Case studies have shown that clinical faculty members are ill equipped to facilitate in these instructional settings.[4] Clinical faculty members further devalued the social sciences in the classroom by teaching decontextualized statistics, upholding inaccurate understandings of race as biological or cultural, and reducing the complexity of social inequalities by focusing on anecdotes of lived experience. I call the latter approach the *anecdotalization effect* because this approach to teaching the social sciences had the effect of delimiting the scale and significance of social inequalities. Dr. Feldman, a white female clinical faculty member, attested to this problem with scale, confiding that the educators at her school did not do students any favors when "we teach them how to pull the baby out of the river, take care of patients one at a time, but we don't teach them how to go upstream and stop whoever is throwing the babies in." She explained that they did not dedicate the time nor did they have the expertise at her school to address the bigger picture. Dr. Li, an Asian clinical faculty member and director of UME, also lamented about faculty members' inability to teach scale, remarking how, "generally speaking, we don't do a great job of teaching that. It's very much about teaching students one-on-one care and not thinking more globally about your community." With limited in-class learning time from experts, clinical faculty members also expressed to students that the *real* learning on social sciences happens in clinical settings—which, as many studies have shown, is a setting where racist, classist, cis- and heteronormative lessons are conveyed.[5]

Presenting a few social scientific facts without the tools for understanding how these outcomes materialized and what the medical profession could do about them confused or frustrated students. Most students described that they did not remember much about what they learned. Recall Caroline, a white female medical student from chapter 5 who could not define "culture" from her medical school coursework, or Riva, a white female medical student from chapter 4, who did not know what she had learned about social inequalities. In both settings, students were given no further explanation of where health and health-care disparities came from and what to do about them. And the students who wanted to learn more—and often pushed back against their schools—were met with indifference or reprimand.

These learning outcomes produced a situation where, as white male medical student, Dylan, mentioned in chapter 5, "no one really cares." Dr. Seery, a white female social scientist at a medical school, explained what she was up against when teaching her students a critical social scientific perspective about understanding human bodies. She echoed Dylan's remarks about how "no one really cares," in saying "for a room full of two hundred people who are in the middle of studying for their gross anatomy, it's harder for them to understand the importance of problems around the body." She continued by describing how "they are being taught, in med school, 95 percent of the time, you need to know this exact structure, and you need to memorize exactly what the structure or function of this thing is." Seery pointed to not only how little time they had to discuss bodies from a critical perspective but also how that limited time and lack of incentives affected students' ability to appreciate the material.

From focusing on skills and the conscripted curriculum to teaching inaccurate information, to students not remembering what they learned or not caring for the material, the included social sciences material seemed merely symbolic, meaningless. But this silence was *productive*: it conferred lessons, but not the lessons the profession dreamed about. When the social sciences were not seen as a body of knowledge with systematically collected data and historically informed understandings of contemporary inequalities but rather as a series of individual-based experiences, it produced dangerous ideological implications. Not teaching about white supremacy is a choice.[6] Therefore, these curricular practices shaped not only student learning outcomes and understandings of inequalities but also perceptions of what was valuable knowledge versus what was just a person's subjective experience.

In the hands of the clinical faculty members, the humanities underwent a slightly different process of knowledge application. The humanities—except for bioethics—were not required at the professional level in the way that the LCME standards demanded an engagement, at least nominally speaking, with the social sciences. At the curricular design phase, clinical faculty members incorporated the humanities in two main formats: trying to admit students who had humanities backgrounds and creating humanities electives that were therapeutic. The former, the *inclusion-as-admissions* approach, created the conditions under which white, Eurocentric, and elite fine arts were celebrated in talent shows; the humanities seemed to be valued for *who* possessed these talents rather than what rigorous study of the humanities could confer. Students viewed these talented peers as effortless in their talents, which was a signal of the "new elite."[7]

The inclusion-as-admissions approach, while directly connected to the profession's past admissions strategy and status quo, was not in line with what humanists and, in some respects, some members of the medical profession envisioned for the humanities in medicine. Although the cathartic value of the humanities has been touted again and again, these arguments have often been part of a far more multifaceted conceptualization of the humanities than simply as stress-reducing leisure.[8] Dr. Morris, a white male humanist, illustrated this sentiment, arguing that "it's crazy to think that the two fields [humanities and medicine] would be separated. They are both the study of the human condition, just approached differently."

Morris went on to say that his literature course "teaches habits and self-reflection. And I think that creates a different type of person. A type of person that I think makes a better doctor. I don't think that books make better doctors. Sitting and talking about books and really thinking about it systematically and learning to consider all types of issues systematically creates people who are more careful in judgment." But this kind of promise of the humanities, as well as what humanists wanted to teach, appeared to be thrown by the wayside to accommodate what clinical faculty members wished to address—or thought could be addressed. Perhaps this was because, as a Latino humanist and clinical faculty member, Dr. Ribeiro, stated, "[T]here is always something about the humanities that is uncomfortable to the medical establishment." Talent shows exhibiting white elite culture did not challenge the status quo; in fact, they celebrated it.

Humanities electives operated with similar principles as the inclusion-as-admissions approach but had an extra lesson of docility attached to them. The elective structure not only continued to center clinical faculty members in their capacity as leading the electives—often on a volunteer basis—but it also affected the content. Clinical faculty members conceptualized the humanities as a set of tools to help them cope with their disorganized, uncertain, and stressful workplace. It was a rather myopic view, where they saw themselves as dealing with burnout, not other health-care workers. Seeing the discontents of their routine clinical work, they reached for the humanities as interpersonal tools aimed at placating the clinician, the patient, and the image of the profession.

It is clear that their concerns about medical student and faculty mental health were valid because the students were not okay. For example, Lisa, a Black female medical student, took a creative writing elective, and she explained that reflective writing assignments were places for students to wrestle with negative emotions that had been stirred up in their learning, She noted, "I started getting very dark." When I asked Riva to tell me more about the goals behind the literature in medicine group she participated in at her school, she gave a jarring example and said rather bluntly, "[T]he main goal was to allow students to know that it's okay to experience a little burnout. It's normal and that they should seek help . . . number two was don't commit suicide, and if you know somebody that might be in danger of committing suicide, tell us, reach out, help this person." She went on to say, "[B]ecause it happened when I was in medical school when I was a first year; there was a second year that committed suicide over Thanksgiving." Thus, while I am critical of the transformation of the humanities into these interpersonal tools of placation—like the humanities as simply journaling—I do not wish to demean the need for therapeutic practices for medical students.

Medical students were not alright, but book clubs were also not the answer because the sources of the stress were not addressed. Instead, students learned to be docile and that it was up to them to figure out how to cope with the miseries of the field, showing how curricular practices were *ideological*. They promoted yet another white elite concept of what it meant to be a professional: one that was "ready and able to work, productively contribute, an atomistic phenomenon bounded and cut off from others, capable, malleable, and compliant."[9] While the responsibility for coping with burnout via book clubs was depicted as lying with the individual, the consequences were conceived to be much bigger: the hospital would lose money, patients would lose trust in the medical profession, there would be a physician workforce shortfall, and so on. A structural problem became individualized and then restructuralized.

The humanities incorporated in these triumphalist and therapeutic ways further limited critique by reinforcing atomization and cultivating status anxiety, on the one hand, and not actually teaching critical approaches to the profession and knowledge, on the other. These curricular failures taught students to avoid advocacy, avoid critique, avoid caring about structural inequalities—all the while teaching students that it would be up to them to learn therapeutic coping strategies to deal with the brutalities that they confronted in their medical training. They were learning communication and coping skills, not knowledge. Medical educators produced curricular injustice and thus reproduced the very inequalities they set out to address.

THE POLITICS OF KNOWLEDGE APPLICATION

Attempts by the U.S. medical profession to engage in UME curricular practices that would produce more humane and equitable physicians have largely failed. The contemporary, physician-centric process of knowledge application produced compounded failure—and the reasons stem from the politics that undergird who was in charge and whose ideas were implemented. Reproduction and contestation are both political acts. This book is therefore about who and what knowledge is for—is knowledge part of an emancipatory project or is it serving an elite agenda? Is knowledge for individual enjoyment and fulfillment, professional or institutional reputation building and status signaling, equity and patient advocacy, or the foundation of applied practice? In thinking through what can be learned from the curricular injustices outlined in this book, we can see the deep entanglement between professional and social identities by focusing on the politics of knowledge application.

Scholars have drawn attention to the broader politics of knowledge that pattern the resources and research agendas of academic actors.[10] They train their analytical eye specifically on the involved institutions that "condition the availability and distribution of power in the production and dissemination of knowledge."[11] The decisions that medical school leaders made around hiring and curricular oversight were political decisions. These decisions put clinical faculty members, who were also mostly white and elite, in positions of curricular power. It was as if they wanted the social sciences without the social scientists, the humanities without the humanists. And it makes sense: with the control over constructing the problems and articulating the solutions, the clinical faculty members control the debate.

I want to remind readers that so far no U.S. professional movements external to the medical profession have mobilized to advance *critical curricular practices*. In other words, the American Sociological Association has not mounted a systematic critique attempting to take the jurisdiction of instructing on the social sciences to medical students, and neither has the Modern Language Association for literature. In addition, I found that the physical proximity of undergraduate schools to the medical school—that is, the availability of faculty and departmental resources in humanities or social sciences disciplines—was not associated with whether the leaders of the medical school chose to engage with them, showing that collaborations between the humanities and social sciences must be cultivated deliberately. Physical proximity alone cannot overpower the political—and organizational—decisions about whose time was rewarded, whose voice was heard, and whose expertise was valued.

As a result of medical school leaders' lack of investment in curricular design and implementation, the responsibility for instruction devolved to individuals. Each part of the knowledge application process generally placed pressure on the individual faculty members involved. First, it fell to the clinical faculty members who had to design the course, then to those who taught, then to the students. But humanities and social sciences faculty members teaching in medical schools felt this responsibility acutely because they did not have a clinical appointment and they were often the only one of their intellectual kind. They felt that the onus was on them to be smart, convincing, and articulate—that the fate of the humanities or social sciences curriculum hinged on their performance and thus not losing students' attention.

Recall Dr. Carley, a white female physician and social scientist, whom we met in the introduction giving an account of her failure. Other medical educators had similar experiences. For example, a white male humanist, Dr. Miller, remarked that had he been "hit by a bus," there would be no discussion of race. Dr. Mogin, a white male social scientist, echoed these sentiments, saying, "[I]f we lose two or three people because they go to another institution that can be our entire capacity." The pressure they felt to do a good job shows that their schools did not have, in Mogin's terms, the "capacity" to support such tasks. Dr. Schumann, a white female clinical faculty member described how the responsibility to design a successful set of curricular practices resided firmly with her. She said, "I feel like I have to prove myself. Because there is only so far that you can go on a leap of faith. I also have to run a program that is actually useful to people here." After claiming that they used many cutting-edge teaching techniques to get students to stay interested, Dr. Geronimos, a white female social scientist, told me, "We're competing with basic science blocks where they have exams every week, and so it's—we have to be on our game."

Dr. Seery explained this pressure to be near-perfect in more detail. She alluded to the tension she and her colleagues felt in undertaking instructional tasks at her school, in discussing how she approached a lecture to the entire cohort of first-year medical students:

> I'm trying to straighten my line. I may think that the economics of the issue are important, I may think the politics of the issue are important, I may think that the history of medical education is important, but if I take too meandering of a path, they're going to get off the sidewalk, and I'm going to be here by myself. But I have colleagues that would tell me that I am wrong. Who think that I just need to figure out a better way to make sure they walk with me on my meandering path. I'm torn sometimes, too. I really want—I feel like if I could just be a better lecturer, then they would get it. If I could just come up with a better example, they would get it. But I am using readings by scholars who I love, who I think are phenomenal at telling the social side to the illness experience, and how physicians can be better. The best that I have found, and it's still not working.

For social scientists or humanists working on medical school faculties where they had limited resources or power, what made them successful—appealing to clinical relevance—sometimes placed an enormous amount of pressure on their own, personal teaching capabilities.[12] As Seery noted, however, she was doing the best she could and it still was not working.

Educators like Seery were up against a behemoth constraint: the clinical faculty members and their interpretive filter. The clinical faculty members held their clinical experience, biomedical knowledge, and prestige in high esteem.[13] While Seery tried to straighten her line, clinical faculty members projected unmerited confidence in tackling these curricular design and implementation tasks that were outside their domain. Other scholars have pointed out how the medical profession normalizes and enculturates confidence in the face of uncertainty, but from this work it also is apparent there are some serious costs.[14] The clinical faculty members' *Hippocratic hubris* has yielded an Icarus moment, but unlike Icarus, the physicians are not the ones who are really bearing the brunt of flying too close to the sun. Wielding curative authority and the clinical experiences that came with it, clinical faculty members taught their students that social inequalities were something they witness in the clinic, not something to study and learn about.[15] They taught them how to perform empathy, fall in line with the status quo, and celebrate white elite culture. In the process of engaging in this curricular work, clinical faculty members protected themselves but not the patients. There is nothing inherently revolutionary about the humanities and social sciences if they are serving the interests of power. Art can pacify; social science can stereotype; physicians can do harm. Knowledge will not automatically save us.[16]

The U.S. medical profession has been engaging in white liberal politics of reform in their process of knowledge application. These curricular practices do not rock the boat. They have a great deal of what legal scholar Derrick Bell calls "interest convergence," where the needs of marginalized groups seem to be addressed because it is convenient for the privileged groups in power, in this case—as in most cases in the United States—white elites. What I have outlined in the book about the process of knowledge application for the medical profession can help explain curricular injustice or reform failure within other institutions, like policing or higher education. It depends at what stage in the process or what part of the process one examines. For example, in a recent California Department of

Justice report on police training practices in the wake of Stephon Clark's murder, they found a "lack of rigor in lesson planning," which denotes a failure at the curricular design level.[17] With institutions of higher education, work on diversity, equity, and inclusion programs have shown that the moral imperative to invest in equity is often replaced by a rationale premised on innovation, which shows how these programs are filtered through similar maintaining-the-status-quo interpretive frames.[18] To draw lessons from this empirical case for other professions or organizations, I will now turn to a discussion of schools that did not perpetuate curricular injustice—to the schools that got it right.

REALIZING THE DREAM:
THE EXCEPTIONS TO THE RULE

Until now, I have largely discussed curricular failures. But educators at a few medical schools were able to realize the profession-wide curricular dreams and deliver on some of the more robust pedagogical promises of the social sciences and humanities. They did so by decentering clinical faculty members and holding students responsible. While it may seem simple, the leaders at these schools hired experts in these fields to design and teach required courses, gave the experts the autonomy to teach the content they wanted, and enforced the importance of this content with an accountability structure. This was an *inclusion-as-integration* approach, where the humanistic and social scientific lessons were deemed foundational to clinical practice and were thus woven into required, expert-led courses. The curricular practices that emanated from these exceptional schools were largely critical. While the courses differed from school to school, students in these courses developed a critical understanding of the social context of their patients, a critical understanding of the medical profession, and a critical understanding of knowledge itself.

One of the central goals that educators espoused at the curricular dreaming phase regarding how to cultivate equitable physicians was for students to be able to contextualize health experiences and health inequalities. Both the social sciences and the humanities could be deployed to realize this promise and could tackle this goal from different angles to show the complexity of human life and the broader structure of inequalities. In one social sciences course at an exceptional medical school, students were evaluated based on their attendance, weekly questions and comments posted to a discussion board, in-class participation, a midterm, and a final paper—akin to a graduate seminar in a social sciences discipline. Within another medical school's "Social and Health Systems" course, "faculty members come from clinical, social science and humanities backgrounds, bringing significant experience in interdisciplinary research and teaching to the seminar session." This course met once a week for ninety minutes.

At another medical school, students were required to take a course on "Essential Knowledge," which was a "concurrent sequence of foundational basic and social sciences courses." First-year students taking the course were "taught the social and population science relevant to the practice of medicine . . . clinical epidemiology, population health, healthcare policy, social medicine, medical ethics, and professionalism." In year 2, this course built on these foundations and "taught students how to think critically about medical knowledge and how to understand the social and political contexts of health and health-care in the United States." In this year 2 seminar, students learned to evaluate the role of health-care providers in achieving health equity as well as explore possible avenues for health-care reform. Pivotal for these courses was the amount of time, content, and faculty expertise.

In yet another course, "Health Systems Science," which took "a broad look at the multiple complex social, environmental and systems factors that impact human health and healthcare in the U.S.," students were explicitly told that it was "vital foundational knowledge essential for the future practice of medicine, regardless of ultimate specialty choice." This emphasis on the essential nature of this content was supported by the format and evaluative structure: "The course is delivered through a combination of lecture, small group discussion and case studies, as well as a flipped classroom model with pre-assigned readings and completion of asynchronous online assignments as well as verbal and written reflection components." These courses were qualitatively different from what most medical schools in my sample provided for students, from the focus on systems and critique to the amount of work that students invested, to the expert instruction, to the amount of time allotted for engagement.

Educators engaged in these critical curricular practices also focused the analytical lens on the medical profession and knowledge itself. According to one course description of a course on race and biomedicine, they began "with an examination of biomedicine as a cultural system and a critical examination of 'culture and cultural competence' to analytically situate the rest of the course matter." In addition, they spent time in the course analyzing "how racial minorities are interpreted and constructed through the lens of medicine." In this course description, what was notable was the commitment to critical examination of the medical profession and its extant interpretive tools. With the case of racism in biomedicine, white male social scientist Dr. Carpano taught the social construction of race in different organ-based lectures at his medical school, saying this embedded approach served as a "corrective to problematic biological conceptions of race."

At another school, where I had the opportunity to interview an educator with a social sciences background and a student, as well as examine the curriculum, the educators described the racist practices that undergirded the developments in biomedical technologies, treatments, and knowledge—everything from the invention of the spirometer to the Tuskegee syphilis study—in their basic and clinical sciences lectures. At another school, where I had a similar data triangulation process, students and faculty members learned concepts such as structural racism, partnering with their school's sociology department in the instruction. These critical approaches were leagues away from other schools where clinical faculty members were teaching, quite literally, the "one drop rule" or a host of other decontextualized, inaccurate, stereotyping, and conscripted curricular injustices.

This critical examination of the profession and knowledge was mirrored in how medical educators also approached the instruction of the humanities at these few exceptional schools. The humanities were not just placating therapeutic tools, nor were they merely vehicles for appreciating white European culture. Dr. Williams, a white male humanist, explained how "many people think that the humanities inquiry in medical education is just about promoting empathy—if that happens, great, but it's much more of a critical undertaking than just that." Dr. Busler, a white female humanist, explained what that critical undertaking could look like. She described a lecture where she taught medical students about critical understandings of the body so that they may better contextualize their work with bodies:

> We start by saying, all right, the body-as-specimen. How does medical education create people who view body in a very particular way, just like parts? Like a med student. They do gross anatomy first. They might be dissecting an arthritic knee, then they see an x-ray of an arthritic knee, then they see slides of what arthritis looks like on a cellular level, and then, in year three, somebody walks into their office with their arthritic knee. So, what is that person going to see? They don't see the arthritic knee embedded into a person. So, body-as-specimen. Then, we talk about body-as-patient. So, like narratives and first-person stories and other ways in which we can learn about the illness experience through art, visual art, or narrative, or storytelling. Then, we do body-as-spectacle. We talk about the metaphors that are associated with abnormal or extraordinary bodies. There are obese bodies, tattooed bodies, or ill bodies. How that might influence not only how people experience their illness, but how physicians then treat those people with those illnesses? How do those three things intersect for a med student when somebody walks through their clinic door?

Compared to much of the therapeutic and triumphalist curricular practices that characterized how the humanities tend to be incorporated in UME, Busler's more critical curricular practices decentered the clinician as the knower and recipient of the humanities' benefits. Instead, the patient—and the type of health care they might need—took center stage.

In another medical school's course description and curricular map, it was evident that, during the first two years of preclinical coursework in the humanities, they required students to complete humanities coursework *every* Tuesday morning. Then, during the third year of clerkships, they required students to describe their rounding experiences and analyze them. Finally, students had to take a four-week immersive humanities course after they finished their clinical rotations in their final year of UME. In a different medical school, students learned from art historians at a local museum whose expertise was valued alongside that of clinical faculty members. Learning a new way to pay attention to detail through a close examination of art, these students learned to improve as diagnosticians and communicators with patients. Students had experts to learn from, readings to do, journal assignments to complete, concepts to apply. As Dr. Gutierrez, a dean of medical education and Latina clinical faculty member, explained, "[T]he delivery of the content is largely about small, structured, sequential lectures with experts who come in and provide the content . . . and there are pieces that students are expected to take back out in a practicum kind of way over the course of three years." She continued, "[S]ometimes it is as explicit as weekly deliverables—this week when you're at the clinic you must do the following three things that will show you the implications of this." Thus, the students were held accountable for learning the concepts by completing homework.

In addition to signaling the importance of the course material by requiring students to do homework, educators also communicated how foundational the knowledge was to future clinical work. As part of the committee that oversaw the development and implementation of the UME curriculum, Dr. Brown, a white male humanist at one medical school, explained, "[W]e try to integrate those issues throughout the curriculum because I think it sends a stronger message if they are taught in anatomy and cardiology and microbiology everything. That this matters for all these things—it is not just that you only have to care about it when you're taking your humanities course." As Brown's example illustrates, clinical relevance *can* encourage the appreciation of critical and structural knowledge, especially if there are experts at the table.

With critical curricular practices, therefore, medical educators wanted to build this knowledge into the conceptual decision-making processes for clinical practice, just as other pieces of biomedical knowledge were integrated. Experts engaged in critical curricular practices insisted on the connection between these subjects and a better delivery of patient care. In addition to having critical content, dedicated curricular time, and homework, medical schools who utilized critical curricular practices also had committed faculty experts to guide their students' acquisition of knowledge (and skills) in the social sciences and humanities.

CAUTIOUS OPTIMISM

Medical students who participated in these critical curricular practices had a much more palpable appreciation for the humanities and social sciences in general and what these fields could do for them as future physicians. They were taught to think; to question; to complain; to subvert; not to be efficient; to get derailed; to wander; to be enthralled; to disrupt; and, perhaps most important, to critique. John, a white male medical student, described why he thought his art course was helpful for him: "I think that the humanities help you get a fuller sense of people—you're caring for patients, you're not caring for robots . . . I think that helps you communicate with and connect with people." While John's remarks could seem like he was just parroting back the curricular dreams as articulated by the medical profession, students were in fact brutally honest and critical of their educational experience. As described in chapter 5, most students reported that they were not taught to think about how the humanities (or social sciences) would improve their future clinical practice.

Charlie, a Latina student I interviewed, also maintained that her coursework in the humanities had strengthened her as a future physician. She took a course on literature in medicine that was modeled after Rita Charon's "Narrative Medicine" program.[19] The course required her to engage in frequent and consistent reflective writing, both about the books and articles the students were reading and how that related to what they were experiencing in the clinic. Charlie recounted:

> I remember my most useful reflection was the first time I had a patient who I knew was going to die. I was the one who sort of diagnosed that he had lung cancer and as a med student you spend a lot of time with a person, so I got close to him. You know, you can get carried away and lost in running from one checkbox to the next. You can sometimes forget that you're dealing with a patient, and that patient can become a set of labs or a set of vital signs.

As students noted with a lot of the humanities content they experienced in their medical education, the reflective writing methods of the "Narrative Medicine" course helped Charlie "build a foundation" for her approach to taking the time to reflect critically on feelings as she grew as a physician.

With the social sciences, students described learning how to approach patients, how to critically evaluate biomedical knowledge, and how to become an advocate for social justice. Evelyn, an Asian female medical student, was required to take a course in her first year on the social foundations of health and health care. She said she learned "to be aware of the community that we are going into, what their socioeconomic status is, and what resources are available to them. That way, we are not telling them 'okay, here's this medication' but we are saying 'okay, this medication might be too expensive for you so let's give you this one.'" She explained how it was clinically essential in coming up with a plan for their health because "we don't just tell them, 'oh yeah, you need to go exercise and walk around the block' when we know that they can't just go walk around the block if there is danger out there." She ended by saying that social scientific *research* was "very valuable in knowing" so she could deliver better health care.

Evelyn highlighted the structural social scientific knowledge as important in contradistinction to simply the anecdotal stories or the communication skills that most medical schools emphasized. Evelyn described being taught to take the patient's social context into account, to pause and see how that might challenge the routines of biomedical advice. She was not just appreciating the anecdotes or stories but rather understanding how, in the context of the United States, there were systematic inequalities that patterned the distribution of resources affecting patient health and health care. In Evelyn's example, health-care access could be difficult, and neighborhoods had different levels of safety. Patrick, a white male medical student, described the purpose of his social sciences block in medical school as helping students to become "more compassionate, educated, and persuasive," to be "champions for the underserved." He explained that *everyone* was implicated in this fight for more equitable health care and that his entire class went to their state's capitol building to learn how to advocate for health care reform.

Expanding on this notion that physicians could be "champions for the underserved" was James, a multiracial male student, who felt that the need for the social sciences extended to both the clinic and beyond after taking a course on the "essentials of social sciences" that was similar to one described above. He noted that "physicians are in a really unique position to advocate for specific policy changes" because they "tend to be very well respected." Here, James voiced a more critical view of the profession and implicated the profession in pursuing change. He went on to say that this position of potential policy influence would be useless if physicians "don't know what the reality is . . . there's no question that there are health disparities by gender identity, by race, and if you don't know what those are and how to fix them then you just perpetuate them." James saw the social sciences as pushing the medical profession to examine critically how they might be complicit in social inequalities and how they might work to address them. These examples illustrate that students who experienced the critical curricular practices came to understand their future role as physicians as fundamentally intertwined with the critical, interpretive, and structural knowledge and skills they learned in the humanities and social sciences.

STRONG INTELLECTUAL INFRASTRUCTURE

Medical school leaders who enacted these critical curricular practices have demonstrated that another way is possible. Curricular injustice is not an inevitable outcome but rather a result of decisions that leaders make in organizing their school, designing their curricular practices, engaging in faculty development, and teaching the courses. To achieve critical curricular practices, medical school leaders must invest in their *intellectual infrastructure*, or the distribution of people and power in a school. A strong intellectual infrastructure is premised on evenly distributed power between humanities and social sciences faculty members, on the one hand, and clinical faculty members, on the other, when it comes to the curriculum—or even the part of the curriculum where the humanities and social sciences are integrated.

Achieving a strong intellectual infrastructure requires the leaders of a medical school to have foresight, be organized, and invest resources. It was clear that Dr. Teatom, a white male social scientist and clinical faculty member, had the type of resources and commitment at his school that could sustain these critical curricular practices. As he explained, "we absolutely insist on having a mixed faculty cohort of clinicians and social science and humanities scholars." Teatom went on to explain how these investments were worth it because they allowed a distribution of power that set the stage for the knowledge to be viewed as having equal epistemological status. It dissolved part of the science/nonscience divide present at most other schools. Describing the benefits of being in an interdisciplinary department, Teatom utilized a biblical metaphor and said, "[I]t's kind of a half ark, there's one of each of us." He continued:

There's so much going on from so many different perspectives that intellectually you're always learning and expanding. I really value that, and one of the things that's great about having such a diverse faculty is that we all teach each other. We meet as a faculty before each class and discuss how we're going to teach the class, what materials we're using. We have a common syllabus, but everybody's free to, you know, add and subtract . . . one of the things that's important about the culture of this department is the idea that nobody is in charge and everybody is charge and nobody's jargon or theoretical approach gets to trump anybody else's. We develop because we have to be intelligible to each other and that the default is "oh, I'm going to learn something new here" rather than "I want to be around people who think like I do."

In outlining his department's approach to curricular design and implementation, Teatom pointed to the commitment to a level epistemological playing field *and* a commitment to continuous learning. This learning happened both with the content that would eventually be taught as well as with discussions around how to organize and distribute the content.

At another school that engaged in critical curricular practices, the dean of UME, Dr. Robinson, a white female clinical faculty member, articulated her approach to enlisting the expertise of nonclinical faculty. She felt that it helped to have a more cohesive vision to incorporating the social sciences. Robinson started by saying how she appointed one or two faculty members who were "responsible for that theme and looking at all the different places it might show up in the curriculum." She explained that "there's all this critique of not calling out specific issues around, for example, race. You want it to be woven in so it's not just 'here's your one-hour of race' but rather it's folded into a lot of the discussions." Robinson continued, "[B]ut it also has to be called out specifically because otherwise, if it's woven in *too* well, then they don't see it." She also showed her understanding of the process of knowledge application: "[S]o the folks who are working on that theme are looking into these issues, like what are the case examples used, how are those examples used, and do they reinforce stereotypes or broaden people's ideas and understandings?" At Robinson's school, they were proactively thinking about how to integrate social scientific knowledge that did not get lost nor reductive. Thus, it was an epistemic and organizational accomplishment when educators were able to incorporate the humanities and social sciences as critical curricular practices.[20]

Funding for the social sciences and humanities faculty members was also helpful here. Elite schools had more financial resources that provided faculty with the ability to produce knowledge and execute goals.[21] Dr. Ribeiro claimed that his school's funding allowed it to "establish a program to organize all of those humanities classes. So that's the infrastructure, now all those classes have a faculty adviser who's there from year to year, who can kind of oversee the continuity." Given that there was a revolving door of clinical faculty members in most schools, the continuity that Ribeiro's school had established helped ensure that there was a more cohesive vision to the course, similar to the way that Robinson's educators approach curricular design.

When it came to the strategy of incorporating the humanities and social sciences as critical curricular practices, these medical schools could invest in hiring scholars, paying for more frequent faculty development, conducting more research on the quality of instructors, sending more educators to conferences, and even funding more pedagogical partnerships with experts. In describing how they were able to get the faculty and facilities for their social sciences department, Dr. Perez, a social scientist at a medical school, said that they were "lucky because [big donor] gave a hundred million dollars to the medical school." The funding, in this sense, was pivotal to the establishment of tenure-track lines for three more scholars in the social sciences department within the medical school. All these capacities help to reinforce the strong intellectual infrastructure around the inclusion of the social sciences.

Compared to some of the frustrations that social sciences and humanities scholars felt at schools that had a weaker intellectual infrastructure, scholars who worked in supportive environments found their work more enjoyable, too. Dr. Carpano, who was a member of both a department of social sciences and a department of medicine, explained the merits of such a position:

> One, it requires me to translate across [social science] and critical frameworks, meaning it requires me to defend what I think is disease really. It also requires me to defend how we come to know health and pathology and biology, and that's the epistemology. Then it requires me to translate that across frameworks so [across] social, philosophical, clinical, biomedical, biogenetic [frameworks] and that is really interesting to me. Then it requires me to also navigate the teacher-student dynamic in ways that [are] really fascinating to me. I mean I wouldn't have spent so much time looking at the medical phenomena if [they] didn't fascinate me.

Carpano was appointed in both his home discipline and the school of medicine. He enjoyed the personal stimulation that having to "speak biomedicine" brought him, but he also thought that these critical curricular practices would have a positive effect on future physicians.

Elite medical schools are much more likely to have critical curricular practices, although not every elite medical school prioritized social sciences and humanities. Some highlighted their biomedical innovation and entrepreneurial capacities. From their opening webpage to their curricular threads, the elite schools that did not have critical curricular practices lauded biomedical research and discovery, individualized treatment innovation and prevention, health-care systems leadership, and customizing the learning experience to the individual student. These elite schools did not have the humanities and social sciences to set them apart from their competitors in their field; instead, they emphasized courses like "Creating Health Care and Life Sciences Ventures" and "Physicians as Leaders" in response to the "rapidly advancing scientific discoveries and emerging innovations in medical technologies." While resources certainly helped, designing and enacting critical curricular practices was therefore a set of deliberate choices by medical school leadership, where they chose to emphasize compassion, critical thinking, and social justice as curricular outcomes.

TOWARD CURRICULAR JUSTICE

Notable exceptions aside, the leaders of medical schools failed to live up to their curricular dreams. Curricular changes will certainly not ameliorate all the social inequalities or fix all the sources of dehumanization in health care in the United States, but leaders of medical schools can implement curricular practices that will better educate future physicians about how to engage in equitable and humane care. The few schools where critical curricular practices are taught bring glimmers of hope and show that leaders of medical schools can move toward curricular justice. I see six central areas in which leaders of medical schools can make concrete improvements: curricular emphases, standard specificity, faculty composition, faculty development, student support, and patient feedback.

The most significant change that leaders of the profession or of medical schools can make would be to shift their curricular emphases. So much of the curricular injustice outlined in this book has to do with educators' placement of the social sciences and humanities and the content that they emphasize. Sociologist Jennifer Mueller notes that "people in power often have the unique capacity and incentive to suppress knowledge and nurture ignorance, not just interpersonally but also by using institutions to structure broad architectures of non-knowledge." Citing Charles W. Mills's work on the racial contract, Mueller contends that "one of the primary ways white people establish allegiance to racial domination is by proving willing to use an epistemology of ignorance to ironically 'misinterpret . . . the world they themselves have made.'"[22] Medical educators cannot ignore critical and structural knowledge about social inequalities; to move toward curricular justice, they must teach medical students these critical curricular practices within the foundational or essential knowledge portion of their curriculum. The equity and empathy problems, whether health and health-care inequalities or patient dissatisfaction, cannot be fixed by educators focusing on the development of communication or coping skills alone.

Once the profession gets the curricular emphases right, they need to add greater specificity to their standards and guidelines. At present, the LCME standards are too ambiguous, and the FRAHME recommendations are merely dawdling as programming suggestions. The AAMC should build up its curricular inventory with sets of recommended readings and test questions that could serve as guides for all medical schools, and more content experts should be involved in this process. The MCAT provides these resources, and these types of resources could serve as a model for the LCME. UK models could also provide inspiration because they supply medical schools with explicit instruction and teaching modules for the social scientific content, with even a decolonization curriculum.[23] Another model could be a medical school that provided an annotated version of the LCME standards where they indicate how to teach critical curricular practices throughout the four years of the UME; for each of the standards contained within LCME Standard 7.6, that medical school offers learning objectives and course materials on their website.

Moving from the profession-wide to the school-specific recommendations, we have already seen how the organizational structures of medical schools tend to place clinical faculty members in positions of curricular power. Thus, their limited understandings of humanities and social sciences content became dominant. Therefore, medical school leaders must invest in diversifying their faculty's disciplinary composition and in building up faculty development. Faculty composition must change along two axes for different reasons. On the one hand, medical school leaders must hire faculty who are not white and not elite—not because their social identities alone confer the kind of expertise needed but because medical schools must actively engage in hiring practices that confront privilege and deemphasize whiteness. On the other hand, leaders must also hire faculty *whose job it is* to teach medical students how to think critically about and engage with dismantling structural inequalities, especially because clinical faculty members have largely failed to show they are able to do so. Understanding racism must be on the same epistemological footing as anatomy if physicians are to provide equitable patient care in the United States.

Of course, building up the faculty is no small feat. If hiring social scientists and humanists is not feasible, then medical schools must invest in curricular development and faculty training. Another potential way in which leaders of medical schools could work to access intellectual resources would be to think about partnering with their undergraduate schools for hiring decisions or cross-listed courses. MD-PhDs who had a PhD in a social science or in the humanities spoke of the flexibility they had as an asset in overcoming epistemic barriers, that their peers would be more likely to listen. Thus, medical schools could invest in augmenting their faculty composition by ramping up MD-PhD training in social sciences and humanities and insist that these tracks be given the same support as basic sciences research tracks, which are powerful moves that a few schools with critical curricular practices have made.

Fifth, students in medical schools confront a host of challenges that may be ubiquitous, or they might be unique to a particular subset of the medical school population. In general, medical school leaders need to examine critically how the structure of medical education may be affecting burnout among their students and how providing optional coursework is only an individual-based solution. In addition to thinking about how they might support students across the board rather than asking them simply to be resilient, I would also recommend that medical school leaders interrogate their curricular practices in relation to how they treat their students from socially marginalized backgrounds. Are they devolving the instruction of social sciences topics onto their students who are from marginalized groups? When students have concerns about the curriculum, how are these concerns handled? If they are going to conscript students to teach, then they should allow them to offer critical feedback on that instruction.

Sixth, for discussions about how to cultivate the ideal physician, one thing that struck me throughout my data collection was that two groups were remarkably absent: the patients and community. As medical school leaders contemplate future curricular change and as they approach the task of cultivating a good physician, they should do a much more thorough job of eliciting and incorporating what their patients and surrounding communities want. Some schools have done a good job at this with their admissions practices, by having community members weigh in and participate during decision-making processes. Thus, while the first four recommendations have to do with suggestions on supporting or facilitating curricular change, the latter two recommendations center on two other groups whose voices are minimized or altogether neglected but nonetheless should be important stakeholders in discussions about moving toward curricular justice.

* * *

It seems trite to say that children are the future, but they are indeed where my hope lies. One of the greatest potentials for change stems from generational cohort replacement. The oldest faculty members trained under a UME curricular structure that was losing its humanities and social sciences because of an influx of biomedicine. The middle generation came of age with very little to no humanities and social sciences instruction, and these debates were largely absent from any sort of medical education discourse. The younger generation of faculty members may have been exposed to discussions and material driving the Institute of Medicine (IOM) report, culturally and linguistically appropriate services (CLAS) act, and LCME standards changes. This is important because most medical school leaders have had no across-the-board immersion in the humanities and social sciences but a ton of clinical experience, and this clinical experience has shaped how they conceptualize the relevance of these subjects. We may see more critical curricular change as younger cohorts gain more leadership positions. Medical graduates who have learned from critical curricular practices and then go on to residencies and academic appointments may be particularly well situated to turn the tide of medical education toward incorporating humanities and social sciences in ways that teach complex critical and interpretive knowledge for clinical practice. The fate of humane and equitable health care should not rest solely on their work, but I am hopeful about students' movements toward curricular justice.

ACKNOWLEDGMENTS

While I do not doubt that I will fail to capture appropriately the extent and tenor of my appreciation for those who have helped make this book happen, this section was a delight to write. I am going to proceed somewhat chronologically, capturing my appreciation of support each step of the way. At the heart of this book are the respondents who made this research possible—I owe an enormous thank you to the medical educators and students who took the time to meet with me and discuss their experiences in designing, teaching, and receiving curricular practices. I am especially grateful to the students and faculty members who have worked and continue to work toward curricular justice at their individual schools and the profession writ large.

I also appreciate the formal and informal research support that facilitated my data collection. I was fortunate to receive grant support from the University of California San Diego (UCSD) Department of Sociology, the UCSD Institute of Humanities, the UCSD Chancellor's Office, the University of California, and the National Science Foundation. I had tremendous informal research support as well. When I traveled to interview medical educators and students or attend conferences, I stayed with many friends to stretch my funding. These friends graciously accepted me into their homes, fed me, lent me their cars or bus passes, and would even print extra consent forms for me at their workplaces. Emma Mintz, Alex Mintz, David Mintz, Kate Lombard, Kelly Robinson, Rachael Ryan, Megan Donovan, Frances Callaghan: thank you for all your help. You gave me so much life, too, during my packed research days.

My research would not have taken the shape it did without the intellectual and thoughtful guidance I received during my doctoral training at UCSD. An immense thank you to John Evans for foregrounding the humanity of research subjects and researchers alike and for imprinting the infamous funnel in my and others' consciousnesses. Thank you, Amy Binder, for giving me a theoretical tool kit and for paying attention to my voice. I also have a deep appreciation for all the feedback and support I received from other members of the department and university: Kwai Ng, Christena Turner, Cathy Gere, Isaac Martin, Danielle Raudenbush, Jeff Haydu, Kevin Lewis, and Andrew Scull. And thank you, Gershon Shafir, for the book's title.

My graduate school friendships were and continue to be a beaming and consistent source of joy, strength, insight, and support for me. A special thank you to Rawan Arar, Lindsay DePalma, and Jane Lilly Lopez for their ongoing inspiration, commiseration, and love. And so many thanks to other dear friends—Kevin Beck, Yao-Tai Li, Pablo Perez-Ahumada, Laura Rogers, Stacy Williams, Jenn Nations, Alexandra Vinson, Davide Carpano, and Haley McInnis—for the comments and the kindness. Beyond my graduate school training, I was lucky to be mentored by a collective of brilliant scholars in my emerging sub-subfield, now officially the Sociology of Health Professions Education Collaborative (SocHPE). Thank you to Alexandra Vinson, Laura Hirshfield, Tania Jenkins, and Kelly Underman—and the rest of the community—for bringing me into the SocHPE fold, embracing my weird, and making my work so much better.

As I moved from graduate student to faculty member, from early drafts to final manuscripts, I have been so fortunate to be part of the Department of Sociology at Temple University. Thank you, Laura Orrico, my fearless writing buddy, for the camaraderie and coffees, and to all the other wonderful faculty members and students who have helped me transform my dissertation into a book: Rebbeca Tesfai, Lu Zhang, Tom Waidzunas, Brian Tuohy, Kevin Loughran, Hana Gebremariam, Andrew Chelius, Olivia Quartey, Megha Gongalla, and Caitlin Tickman. I am also incredibly grateful to the support from Kim Goyette and Dustin Kidd, as well as Temple University's Liberal Arts Undergraduate Research Award, Summer Research Award, and pre-tenure sabbatical, for helping me have protected time to finish writing this book.

My book would not be in its present form were it not for the incredible support from Columbia University Press and most notably Eric Schwartz. I could not have asked for a more calm, insightful, and optimistic guide to usher me through the process of writing a book for the first time. Thank you to the readers of the proposal and manuscript for such thoughtful and constructive feedback. And thank you to my developmental editor, Audra Wolfe, for helping me tackle the readers' suggestions and re-envision the processual organization of the book. Of course, all the book's limitations are my own.

A final set of remarks are due to my nears and dears, those who maintained my sense of self and tolerated my frequent absences because I was "working on my book." To Lauren Mayberry, Mark Wright, Chris Anderson, Anna Andersen, Kiki Kalkstein, Daniel DuBois, Jill Allenbaugh, the Marlborough Street Crew, the Andersens, the Engles, the Robinsons, the Mintzes, the Wrights, the Olsens, and the Froneks: you all have given me far more than I deserve. To Alanna Beroiza, thank you for going down any and every rabbit hole with me. To Emma Mintz, thank you for caring about the historical context and (never) believing in me. To Mike Rispoli, thank you for your multitudes and your hype. To Mom and Dad, thank you for being the kinds of physicians that I believe physicians should be and for your lifelong support of my pursuit of a career that I found to be important. To Lindsay, thank you for your hilarity, your sweetness, and our closeness. And, finally, to my grandparents, thank you for believing in me with such fierce confidence and for supplying me with chocolates. While I feel grateful to so many people—and for so many reasons—for getting to have the opportunity to pursue this professorial path, one of the best parts of it all was the time I spent living with my grandparents throughout graduate school.

METHODOLOGICAL APPENDIX

DATA SOURCES AND RESEARCH DESIGN

When I designed this project in 2015, other scholars' methodological appendixes were instrumental in helping me envision how to carry out a research project of my own. Therefore, I describe here, in as much detail as possible, the decisions I made in designing and collecting data for this project. While I present mostly interview data in the book, my analysis also drew on data from profession-wide and individual-school-level reports, publications, and conferences. I first describe the interview data with medical educators and students; then I outline the observational, curricular, and organizational data; and I conclude with a discussion of my analytical strategy and my project's limitations.

INTERVIEW DATA

Between 2015 and 2017, I conducted ninety semistructured interviews with U.S. medical educators and students about how they conceptualized the value of the humanities and social sciences, how they viewed the purpose of these sets of knowledge for medicine, and how they perceived the various challenges and opportunities they confronted when attempting to include these bodies of knowledge into their undergraduate medical education (UME) curriculum.

These interviews gave me an account of successes and failures, and they also illuminated how these clinical faculty members, humanities and social sciences faculty members, and students defined the relevance of these fields for medicine. I interviewed sixty medical educators: thirty with a clinical (MD) background and thirty with a humanities or social sciences (PhD/EdD) background, and thirty students from thirty-seven different medical schools.

My sample of medical educators included faculty in senior leadership positions, UME program directors, and teaching faculty who had direct control or responsibility for curricula in the first four years of medical school. Of the sixty educators interviewed, thirty-six held at least an MD degree (eight held an MD-PhD, with a PhD in either a humanities [one], social science [five], or biomedical discipline [two]). An additional eleven held just a PhD in a humanities discipline, ten held just a PhD in a social science, and three others held an EdD with extensive postgraduate training in the humanities. These scholars with humanities and social sciences backgrounds taught in medical schools, like the medical educators with MDs; therefore, I often referred to both groups as "educators" when I was describing something that all educators reported or faced. I referred to the MDs as clinical faculty members.

My central objective for interviewing people from these three groups was to leverage comparisons across fields (e.g., clinical, humanities, social sciences) and across status (e.g., faculty or student). I used the same interview guide with each medical student and an expanded version of that guide with educators. I asked the educators to describe how and why they became involved and interested in medical education, how they approached curricular design, why they wanted to include the humanities and social sciences in their curriculum, how they persuaded their colleagues and students of the importance of their developed courses, what reservations they had about the inclusion of these types of knowledge, what evidence best illustrated the success of a course, what students gained most from the course, and the rewarding and challenging parts of the incorporation process. Instead of asking students about curricular development, I asked them about curricular reception and to reflect on how the courses were structured, what they read, how they were evaluated, and their impressions of these courses. At the close of all the interviews, I asked respondents if—and if so, how—they thought these curricular practices made students into better physicians. The interviews lasted between twenty-six and seventy-two minutes, with an average length of fifty-one minutes. All the interviews were transcribed from audio to text, except for five interviews because the participants declined to be recorded.

Recruitment and Sampling

I began the project by identifying potential respondents through medical school websites and at professional conferences where discussions about the inclusion of humanities and social sciences for UME occurred. I emailed potential respondents at schools in a particular geographical area; I chose locations where there were either many medical schools in the metropolitan area or the schools were within three to four hours of travel by car, train, or bus. I would email every person who met the inclusion criteria as medical educators (PhDs, MDs, and EdDs) at each of the institutions in that geographical area. My inclusion criteria for medical educators, which I describe in greater detail in the sections below on each of the type of respondents, was identifiable on each school's website because I could access the potential respondent's curriculum vitae (CV), which let me know their degree, year of graduation, and current and past positions at the medical school.

While educators' contact information was listed on websites, medical students' contact information was not. Therefore, I engaged in snowball sampling with medical students. First, I contacted medical students through my personal network of friends and family members. Once I conducted an interview with a medical student, I would create a snowball chain, ultimately creating many small chains. In addition, I met potential respondents at professional meetings and workshops. While I spoke to a student and an educator at the same medical school for most of my sample, there were some schools in which I did not yield a match. In total, I interviewed students and educators from thirty-seven schools.

My respondents' gender identities were consistent with the cis-normative dominance of the gender binary in medical education.[1] I interviewed fifteen male students, fifteen female students, thirty-two male educators, and twenty-eight female educators. The educator ratio mirrored broader trends in medical school faculties, where women were underrepresented; however, my sample might actually overstate the degree to which female faculty members hold positions of leadership in medical schools.[2] Regarding racial composition, the educators were largely white, which also mirrored broader trends in medical school and academic faculties; of the sixty educators, only eight identified as persons of color.[3] The medical students in my study exhibited more racial diversity, with fifteen identifying as white and fifteen identifying as students of color—as mostly Black, Latinx, or multiracial. By virtue of my snowball sampling strategy, my sample overstated the representation of students of color. I did not ask respondents about their sexual orientation or class position, although some volunteered that information.

Interviews with Clinical Faculty Members

Clinical faculty members divided their time along the tripartite mission of medical education: teaching, research, and clinical work. First, within the teaching part of the medical school's foci, there was the MD program, which existed adjacent to other degree-granting professional programs, like MPH- or PhD-granting graduate programs at medical schools. This education branch of the medical school oversaw UME, graduate medical education (GME), and continuing medical education (CME). Depending on the school, the UME branch included various offices and groups. At some schools, there was a department of medical education; however, most U.S. medical schools had something like an office of medical education, with deans and coordinators who advised students and faculty members regarding the development, implementation, and evaluation of the UME curricular practices.

Depending on the school, the office of medical education took on other responsibilities, such as community engagement; student affairs; and/or diversity, equity, and inclusion. Some medical schools organized their UME students into learning communities, which had a program coordinator who was responsible for overseeing the faculty members leading small groups and for addressing student concerns about their learning. At all schools—regardless of whether there were learning communities—there were course directors for various sequences within the preclinical (first eighteen to twenty-four months of medical school) and clerkship (final twenty-four to thirty months of medical school) years. These sequences entailed a mixture of instruction in the basic sciences (e.g., microbiology), social sciences (e.g., anthropology), clinical sciences (e.g., anatomy), humanities (e.g., literature), and practice of medicine (e.g., interviewing a patient).

Second, for the research wing of medical schools, various departments conducted basic science or applied clinical research. Some (roughly 10 percent) of the faculty members who taught medical students were pulled from these departments (e.g., biochemistry). These faculty members had less sustained engagement with medical students because students rotated through curricular topics so quickly, spending just four to six weeks on a particular basic sciences topic. Third, for the clinical practice dimension of medical schools, some clinical faculty members taught, advised, and led students when they were doing their clinical rotations. The amount of time clinical faculty members spend with patients varies depending upon the percentage of their time that they have dedicated to clinical service. Clinical faculty members comprised the bulk of all full-time positions at U.S. medical schools, at roughly 89 percent.

I conducted thirty in-depth, semistructured interviews with clinical faculty members. Inclusion criteria for these medical educators were based on their intellectual, administrative, or professional contribution to medical education, on the one hand, and their medical school, on the other. To meet the former criterion, the clinical faculty members must have had some formal involvement with curricular development, evaluation, implementation, coordination, facilitation, or instruction, although they did not have to identify this work as their primary academic or professional objective. To meet the latter criterion, the educator must have been appointed within an accredited MD-granting school. The interviews allowed the "official" arbiters of UME dreaming, design, and implementation to describe how they developed and evaluated curricular practices, why they wanted (or did not want) to include the humanities and social sciences, and what these bodies of knowledge meant to them.[4] They were also able to explain some of the challenges and opportunities that affected the incorporation of the humanities and social sciences into their UME curriculum, describing the curricular practices that they would ideally have had compared to the curriculum they were able to implement, and the discrepancies that arose between the two.[5]

Interviews with Humanities and Social Sciences Scholars

I conducted fifteen in-depth, semistructured interviews with humanities scholars (twelve with a PhD in a humanities field, three with an EdD and extensive training in the humanities) and fifteen interviews with social sciences scholars (all with a PhD) who were involved with UME curricular practices. The rationale for interviewing equal amounts of humanities and social sciences scholars involved in medical education was because I wanted to disentangle the two areas of knowledge application; see where they intersected, collaborated, and disagreed; and ultimately understand these scholars' separate and joint degrees of success in implementing their fields into medical education.

Inclusion criteria for these humanities and social sciences scholars were based on their intellectual, administrative, or professional contributions to medical education, which was similar to the inclusion criteria for clinical faculty members. Because most of these faculty cannot practice as clinicians, their employment took on different shapes: sometimes they held an appointment in a medical school; other times they were joint or courtesy appointments. Practically speaking, this sample included scholars who taught medical students but also undergraduate students, scholars who taught solely medical students, and scholars who designed curriculum for medical students and oversaw courses. Thus, at a minimum, these scholars had a tangible relationship to medical students at their school. Some were also engaged in research on medical education; however, that was not required. The curricular practices that these scholars tended to be involved in varied by school; however, these humanities and social sciences scholars' main curricular engagement occurred mostly in either teaching foundational courses in their discipline, lecturing in or facilitating a practice of medicine (POM) sequence course on the "how to doctor" part of medicine, or leading elective programming in their discipline or a variety of humanities and social sciences disciplines.

Most scholars I spoke with were in their positions either accidentally or as a backup plan. The interviews allowed the "official" knowledge producers to describe how they defined their fields, conceptualized their curricular interventions, and understood their role—and the role of their knowledge—in medical education.[6] The interviews also gave scholars the space to explain what difficulties they encountered in implementing their curricular practices, describe the work that they would ideally have done compared to the work that they were able to do, and name the discrepancies that arose between the two.[7] I also asked them to consider the contributions of their discipline to the profession of medicine.

Interviews with Medical Students

I conducted thirty in-depth, semistructured interviews with medical students to understand how the consumers of medical education valued—and absorbed—the humanities and social sciences for future clinical practice. Inclusion criteria for these students was based on their enrollment at a medical school and their completion of a component of the curriculum with humanistic or social scientific material. The interviews allowed the "official" consumers of UME curricular practices to describe how they received them, what they found to be the relevant features of the humanities and social sciences in their training, and what this knowledge meant to them. Students were also able to situate these curricular practices within their broader training.[8]

With the interviews portion of the project, my position was relevant in three central ways: my status as a student; my status as a white, cisgender woman; and my status as a child of physicians. For my status as a graduate student at the time of data collection, most educators viewed me as a student they could explain things to, whereas most students saw me as a peer. Students were very open about the difficulties of their educational path. My position as a white, cisgender female was important for the context of the in-person interview with both participants of color and white participants. I believe that my questions about the curriculum (e.g., how race was taught and whether racism was taught) signaled my concern about how race holds powerful social meanings and consequences in U.S. society.[9] With white students and educators, I had to ask many iterations of the question about how matters of race were taught in their medical school; with faculty members and students of color, I did not need to reformulate this type of question repeatedly. I leveraged my cultural capital as a child of physicians as much as I could when conducting interviews and generally felt comfortable with the Hippocratic hubris that many clinical faculty members seemed to possess.

OBSERVATIONAL DATA

To supplement the interview data, I engaged in nonparticipant observation to better understand the nature and purpose of the humanities and social sciences in UME, along with the opportunities and challenges related to these fields at the profession-wide level.[10] These observations occurred at scientific, pedagogical, and professional conferences like the Association of American Medical Colleges (AAMC) annual meeting. I attended this meeting three years in a row, 2015 to 2017. These conferences had around 1,800 medical educators in attendance. Attendees held varying degrees (e.g., MD, PhD, EdD, MedD, MA, MPH) in a variety of fields (e.g., biomedicine, basic sciences, social sciences, humanities, education). In addition, they held varying degrees of power in their medical school (e.g., deans, associate deans, professors, clinical/adjunct professors, residency coordinators, UME coordinators, residents, and medical students). Subsections included regional, UME, GME, CME, medical education scholarship, student affairs, educational affairs, information technology, and dean groups.

The AAMC annual meeting featured the latest curricular developments. The sessions throughout the day varied in content and length. There were relatively fewer concurrent panels compared to the American Sociological Association's annual meeting. The six central formats for the sessions were: (1) "update" by a professional leader about the latest standard, particular finding, or proceedings from a meeting; (2) paper presentation and discussion of one preselected paper that was a review paper of a particular topic in medical education; (3) a workshop where a number of educators presented briefly on a topic and then had the audience members engage in an exercise to teach them how the presentation was relevant to medical education and how to use it in their own educational efforts and research; (4) a panel with three papers and a discussant; (5) a business meeting for a particular organizational body; and (6) a reception of a subgroup or the entire AAMC medical education meeting attendees. I downloaded the PowerPoint slides from the talks, took notes during my observation, and completed field notes when I returned home. I found this data to be illustrative of many findings I uncovered throughout the course of my interviews, and I remain astounded that these meetings provided so much free coffee and food for participants!

CURRICULAR AND ORGANIZATIONAL DATA

I wanted to understand the broader professional field to help contextualize my interviews and observations, so I also gathered curricular and organizational data. To identify an exhaustive set of accredited, MD-granting schools in the United States, I first used the medical school members list on the AAMC website, which contained the addresses and websites of each of these schools. Then, I cross-referenced this list with the accredited MD programs in the United States list on the Liaison Committee on Medical Education (LCME) website. I downloaded the LCME list and created a spreadsheet in Excel, where each school constituted a row; I deleted schools from the analysis that were in the process of becoming accredited because they were newly formed schools or newly brought under the jurisdiction of the LCME (e.g., Kaiser Permanente School of Medicine in Pasadena, California; San Juan Bautista School of Medicine in San Juan, Puerto Rico). The final list for this project consisted of 137 schools.

Before I gathered any data, I visited the websites of the schools where I had interviewed faculty members and students because I had a better idea of their curricular practices. With this preliminary investigation of these schools, I began outlining the types of curricular information that would potentially be available. Course descriptions and curricular maps were the most reliably available. While every single medical school had a website, they varied in their navigational organization and amount of content. In general, they all contained information about the history of the school; the school's leadership and administration; the school's mission and diversity statements; the admissions procedures and requirements; the research facilities and foci; the clinical and other discipline departments; the centers, institutes, and programs; the students' resources; and the curricular practices. Not every medical school's website listed which faculty members were teaching which courses, so I did not systematically gather that information for every school.

After viewing course descriptions and curricular maps, I gathered every piece of available data pertaining to the curricular requirements and electives. Sometimes this entailed copying and pasting the information from the website into a Word document; other times, I downloaded the PDF attachments featured on the website. The approach that the school took to organizing the information on the website patterned how easily I could access this information; some schools placed the information on curricular requirements under "Students" in their navigation, others under "Academics," and still others under "Department of Medical Education." Sometimes information about electives was listed under the "Centers" tab; other times, it was featured with the information on curricular requirements. Sometimes it was listed with the curriculum, or it was listed under "Student Life," "Student Affairs," or "About" and contained in either a brochure for prospective students or a student manual or handbook for current students.

I report some of these curricular data in table A.1. It is important to note that these numbers reflected what schools reported on their websites or what I identified through interviews and observations in 2015 to 2017; therefore, these numbers might not reflect present

TABLE A.1 ORGANIZATIONAL FEATURES AND CURRICULAR DATA

Organizational Feature	Codes	Raw (N = 137)	Percentage
Type	Private	53	38.7
	Public	84	61.3
Location	Urban	85	62
	Rural/suburban	52	38
Intellectual resources			
Proximity to undergraduate	No affiliation	23	16.8
	Not close	43	31.4
	Close	71	51.8
Research centers	No social sciences or humanities	50	36.5
	Center for social sciences	52	38
	Center for humanities	13	9.5
	Centers for social sciences and humanities	22	16
Departments	No social science nor humanities	105	76.7
	Department of social sciences	24	17.5
	Department of humanities	5	3.6
	Departments for social sciences and humanities	3	2.2
Dean representation			
Professional	MD	120	87.6
	PhD (biomedical)	6	4.4
	MD-PhD	11	8
Social	White male	105	76.7
	White female	19	13.9
	Male of color	10	7.3
	Female of color	3	2.2
Student representation	Less than 13% students of color	91	66.4
	Between 13% and 26%	37	27.0
	More than 26%	9	6.6
Curriculum	Critical curricular practices	14	10.2
(Not mutually exclusive)	Shoehorned social sciences	127	92.7
	Elective in humanities*	113	82.5
	Small-group instruction on social topics†	104	75.9
Research	Required	41	29.9
	Optional	96	70.1
Community service	Required	52	38
	Optional	85	62

* Suggestive of therapeutic curricular practices.
† Suggestive of conscripted curricular practices.

curricular patterns. They also captured what schools said—which, as my book showed, a school's or profession's curricular discourse was not the same as their curricular actions. I also gathered publicly available information about the organizational features of each medical school to get a better sense about the landscape of schools. I examined school type, location, proximity to the undergraduate campus, distribution of research centers and departments, dean representation by professional and social identity, and student representation by social identity. With the exception of school type (private or public), location (urban or rural/suburban), all the other features are subject to change as medical schools expand; research centers and departments are created, merged, or dissolved; deans change; and new students are admitted.

I am including this data in the methodological appendix to show the full research process because I ultimately did not have conclusive data about curricular patterns based on these organizational features. Yes, schools with more resources were more likely to have strong intellectual infrastructure to incorporate the humanities and social sciences as critical curricular practices. But the resources alone did not guarantee a commitment to that approach because some of the schools with more resources poured their financial resources into entrepreneurial endeavors (e.g., business strategy and patent law) as opposed to incorporating critical lessons from the social sciences and humanities.

Despite these differences between medical schools, and the many educators claiming that "if you've seen one medical school, you've seen one medical school," I found that the overwhelming presence of clinical faculty members and their interpretive lens rose above these organization-level distinctions. The dominance of the clinical faculty at medical schools was the main story.

ANALYTIC STRATEGY

After gathering all these data, I identified the structure, objectives, explanations, and impacts of the inclusion of the humanities and social sciences in medical education. I remained interested in the mismatch between talk and action. With the curricular, organizational, and observational data, I situated the successes; failures; constructions of the relevance of humanistic and social scientific knowledge for medicine; and negotiations of interdisciplinary work within the broader social, cultural, interprofessional, and organizational environment. With the interviews, I identified contemporary conceptualizations of the value of the humanities and social sciences for clinical practice, the challenges and opportunities that educators from different fields faced in attempting to collaborate in the implementation of these bodies of knowledge into medical education, and the overall impressions of the success and failure of their attempts.

I uploaded all texts, field notes, and interviews into Dedoose software for Mac computers and stored everything in a secure, password-protected computer. In compliance with human research protection protocol, I kept the identifying information about participants and their affiliated schools confidential—and used pseudonyms and generalized language to discuss the respondents and their schools in the book. I used the field notes as supplementary memos and did not code them systematically. I coded and recoded all interview and curricular material, tagging specific excerpts and then aggregating codes. My coding was inspired by grounded theory and was done in an iterative and reciprocal process of deduction and induction—deductive codes were based on theoretical interests (e.g., positivistic social sciences, epistemic hostility) and inductive codes were generated from patterns in the data (e.g., burnout, clinical relevance, student labor).

For the inductive codes, initial coding with the interview data was line by line, where I focused on words that reflected action, specifically gerunds (e.g., "branding," "developing," "resisting," "describing," "discussing," "valuing," "devolving").[11] Then, I would think about what processes were occurring and whether there were any tacit assumptions and sequencing at work (e.g., "depicting the humanities as part of the school's brand," "describing the students as pivotal to the instruction of social science," "devolving the responsibility for well-being onto students themselves"). Therefore, I focused my analysis on explicating the implicit actions and meanings in the enactment of curricular practices at each stage of the process of knowledge application.

LIMITATIONS

There were limitations to my data collection that constrained what I could claim. First, with regard to the interview data, there was the potential for self-selection bias. My sample may represent the more enthusiastic supporters of the integration of the humanities and social sciences into medical education, precisely because they were the ones who agreed to participate in an interview about that process. With the supplemental profession-wide and curricular data—and because I found so many limitations to their enacted curricular practices—I believe that I was still able to capture accurately the ways in which these curricular practices operated in UME. I think that my finding that a rare few were able to achieve critical curricular practices, despite many more wanting to do it, was even more striking.

Second, my small sample of students limited the degree to which my findings represent experiences of students at all medical schools; however, work by students and medical educators analyzing their particular medical schools seems to corroborate many of my findings.[12] Third, my corpus of data was limited to MD-granting schools. I excluded doctor of osteopathy (DO) from the analysis because I already had so many variables to consider. DO schools, however, have a more holistic tradition compared to MD schools, so it is possible that more of these schools had critical curricular practices. These schools tend to have less funding, less prestige, and less personnel[13]—that is, less intellectual infrastructure—so at the same time, I believe that it would be unlikely to have seen critical curricular practices in abundance at these institutions.

Finally, and this is a limitation I take very seriously, my data focused on what students learned, not how they practiced. UME is just one phase in a long series of educational experiences that physicians will undergo. The decision to teach visual diagnostic skills with art, the decision not to instruct students about the social construction of race in a didactic setting, or the decision to provide students with a therapeutic book club—all could have different effects on actual clinical practice. While my respondents articulated reservations about the long-standing effects of these curricular practices, I think that some of the most supportive statements that buttress the longer-term impacts of these curricular practices came from the medical educators and students who had clinical experience and could see how what they learned in UME materialized in their clinical practice. In addition, research from other scholars also supports the claim that these curricular injustices have the potential to have a negative impact on patient care.[14]

I cannot capture everything with these data, but it is my hope that what I do capture is informative. And I hope my work provides ample opportunities for future researchers to pick up where I left off.

NOTES

INTRODUCTION

1. Dr. Carley is a pseudonym. I use pseudonyms for all my study respondents.
2. Christina Amutah et al., "Misrepresenting Race—The Role of Medical Schools in Propagating Physician Bias," *New England Journal of Medicine* 384, no. 9 (2021): 872–878.
3. Alice O'Connor, *Poverty Knowledge: Social Science, Social Policy, and the Poor in Twentieth-Century U.S. History* (Princeton, NJ: Princeton University Press, 2001); Louise Seamster and Victor Ray, "Against Teleology in the Study of Race: Toward the Abolition of the Progress Paradigm," *Sociological Theory* 36, no. 4 (2018): 315–342.
4. David Skorton and Ashley Bear, *The Integration of the Humanities and Arts with Sciences, Engineering, and Medicine in Higher Education: Branches from the Same Tree* (Washington, DC: National Academy of Sciences, 2018).
5. Skorton and Bear, *The Integration of the Humanities and Arts with Sciences, Engineering, and Medicine.*
6. The World Health Organization's tenet of *social accountability* mandates that medical educators prioritize the needs of the populations they serve: "It is proposed, therefore, that social accountability for medical schools be defined as the obligation to direct their education, research and service activities towards addressing the priority health concerns of the community, region, and/or nation they have a mandate to serve." Charles Boelen and Jeffrey E. Heck, *Defining and Measuring the Social Accountability of Medical Schools* (Geneva: World Health Organization, 1995), 3.
7. Liaison Committee on Medical Education (LCME), *Functions and Structure of a Medical School: Standards for Accreditation of Medical Education Programs*

Leading to the MD Degree (Washington, DC: Association of American Medical Colleges, 2018).

8. LCME, *Functions and Structure of a Medical School*; N. Bostick, K. Morin, R. Benjamin, and D. Higginson, "Physicians' Ethical Responsibilities in Addressing Racial and Ethnic Healthcare Disparities," *Journal of the National Medical Association* 98, no. 8 (2006): 1329–1334.

9. They also published a monograph, guidebook, and professional development program, stating that these fields were integral to medical education.

10. David J. Doukas, Lawrence B. McCullough, and Stephen E. Wear, "Reforming Medical Education in Ethics and Humanities by Finding Common Ground with Abraham Flexner," *Academic Medicine* 85, no. 2 (2010): 318–323.

11. Sarah Berry, Therese Jones, and Erin Lamb, "Editors' Introduction: Health Humanities: The Future of Pre-Health Education Is Here," *Journal of Medical Humanities* 38 (2017): 353–360.

12. Association of American Medical Colleges, "Diversity in Medical Education: Facts and Figures 2016," vol. 6, *Facts and Figures Report* (Washington, DC: AAMC, 2016).

13. Samuel W. Bloom, "Structure and Ideology in Medical Education: An Analysis of Resistance to Change," *Journal of Health and Social Behavior* 29, no. 2 (1988): 294–306; Lauren B. Edelman, "Legal Ambiguity and Symbolic Structures: Organizational Mediation of Civil Rights Law," *American Journal of Sociology* 97, no. 6 (1992): 1531–1576; Timothy Hallett and Marc Ventresca, "Inhabited Institutions: Social Interactions and Organizational Forms in Gouldner's Patterns of Industrial Bureaucracy," *Theory and Society* 35, no. 2 (2006): 213–236; Katherine C. Kellogg, *Challenging Operations: Medical Reform and Resistance in Surgery* (Chicago: University of Chicago Press, 2011); Donald W. Light, "Toward a New Sociology of Medical Education," *Journal of Health and Social Behavior* 29, no. 3 (1988): 307–322.

14. Anthropologists would also document their trials and tribulations in incorporating their material into the curricular practices of medical schools. See Robin F. Bagdley and Samuel W. Bloom, "Behavioral Sciences and Medical Education: The Case of Sociology," *Social Science and Medicine* 7, no. 1 (1973): 923–941; Byron Good and Mary-Jo DelVecchio Good, "Disabling Practitioners: Hazards of Learning to Be a Doctor in American Medical Education," *American Journal of Orthopsychiatry* 59, no. 3 (1989): 303–321; Richard G. Petersdorf and A. R. Feinstein, "An Informal Appraisal of the Current Status of 'Medical Sociology,'" in *The Relevance of Social Science in Medicine*, ed. Leon Eisenberg and Arthur Kleinman (Dordrecht: Reidel, 1981), 27–45.

For a more recent account, see Warwick Anderson, "Teaching Race at Medical School: Social Scientists on the Margin," *Social Studies of Science* 38, no. 5 (2008): 785–800.

15. Bloom, "Structure and Ideology in Medical Education," 294.

16. Howard Waitzkin, *Politics of Medical Encounters: How Patients and Doctors Deal with Social Problems* (New Haven, CT: Yale University Press, 1991); Howard Waitzkin, "Changing Patient-Physician Relationships in the Changing Health-Policy Environment," in *Handbook of Medical Sociology*, ed. C. Bird, P. Conrad, and A. Fremont (Upper Saddle River, NJ: Prentice-Hall, 2000), 271–283.

17. Light, "Toward a New Sociology of Medical Education."

18. John W. Meyer and Brian Rowan, "Institutionalized Organizations: Formal Structure as Myth and Ceremony," *American Journal of Sociology* 83, no. 4 (1977): 340–363.

19. Edelman, "Legal Ambiguity and Symbolic Structures;" Frank Dobbin and Alexandra Kalev, "Architecture of Inclusion: Evidence from Corporate Diversity Programs," *Harvard Journal of Law and Gender* 30, no. 2 (2007): 279–301.

20. Hallett and Ventresca, "Inhabited Institutions;" Amy J. Binder, "Why Do Some Curricular Challenges 'Work' While Others Do Not? The Case of Three Afrocentric Challenges: Atlanta, Washington DC, and New York State," *Sociology of Education* 73, no. 1 (2000): 69–91; Amy J. Binder, *Contentious Curricula: Afrocentrism and Creationism in American Public Schools* (Princeton, NJ: Princeton University Press, 2002).

21. Kellogg, *Challenging Operations.*

22. Diane Vaughan outlines how organizational practices can encourage or produce the normalization of deviance: "mistake, mishap, and disaster are socially organized and systematically produced by social structures . . . embedded in the banality of organizational life and facilitated by an environment of scarcity and competition, elite bargaining, uncertain technology, incrementalism, patterns of information, routinization, organizational and interorganizational structures, and a complex culture." This functional incoherence in organizations has been described by Cohen et al. (1972) as "organized anarchies." Diane Vaughan, *The Challenger Launch Decision: Risky Technology, Culture, and Deviance at NASA* (Chicago: University of Chicago Press, 1996), xiv; Michael D. Cohen, James G. March, and Johan P. Olsen, "A Garbage Can Model of Organizational Choice," *Administrative Science Quarterly* 17, no. 1 (1972): 1–25.

23. Elizabeth Popp Berman, "Explaining the Move Toward the Market in US Academic Science: How Institutional Logics Can Change Without Institutional Entrepreneurs," *Theory and Society* 41, no. 3 (2012): 261–299; Elizabeth Popp Berman, "Not Just Neoliberalism: Economization in US Science and Technology," *Science, Technology and Human Values* 39, no. 3 (2014): 397–431; Frank Donoghue, *The Last Professors: The Corporate University and the Fate of the Humanities* (Bronx, NY: Fordham University Press, 2008); Edward J. Hackett et al., eds., *The Handbook of Science and Technology Studies* (Cambridge, MA: MIT Press, 2008); Louis Menand, *The Marketplace of Ideas: Reform and Resistance in the American University* (New York: Norton, 2010).

24. Regarding the "care work," scholars have shown that those from the "softer" disciplines within the social sciences and humanities were put in positions of caring for science, technology, engineering, mathematics, and medicine (STEMM) fields "by learning how to observe, protect, and communicate without disturbing technical or professional boundaries." Ana Viseu, "Caring for Nanotechnology? Being an Integrated Social Scientist," *Social Studies of Science* 45, no 5 (2015): 645. Recent research on the relationships between biomedical and humanistic scholars depict a relationship filled with tension, inequity, and even hostility: Des Fitzgerald et al., "Ambivalence, Equivocation and the Politics of Experimental Knowledge: A Transdisciplinary Neuroscience Encounter," *Social Studies of Science* 44, no. 5 (2014): 453–473; Paul Rabinow and Gaymon Bennett, *Designing Human Practices: An Experiment with Synthetic Biology* (Chicago: University of Chicago Press, 2012). In their work with molecular biologists, cultural anthropologists Rabinow and Bennett found that, despite their conversational expertise and eagerness to learn more about molecular biology, "no reciprocity emerged, nor was it encouraged" from their colleagues. Describing the failure of their collaborative endeavors, Rabinow and Bennett explain that they did not sacrifice the frankness of their speech; in contrast, sociologist Fitzgerald and colleagues (p. 716) noted that they practiced "reticent politesse" with their biomedical collaborators, refraining to speak out and living with the feelings of discomfort and uncertainty in order to help the collaboration occur more successfully. See also Mathieu Albert, Elise Paradis, and Ayelet Kuper, "Interdisciplinary Promises Versus Practices in Medicine: The Decoupled Experiences of Social Sciences and Humanities Scholars," *Social Science and Medicine* 126, no. 1 (2015): 17–25; Fitzgerald et al., "Ambivalence, Equivocation and the Politics of Experimental Knowledge;" Rabinow and Bennett, *Designing Human Practices*; Viseu, "Caring for Nanotechnology?;" Andrew S. Balmer et al.,

"Taking Roles in Interdisciplinary Collaborations: Reflections on Working in Post-ELSI Spaces in the UK Synthetic Biology Community," *Science and Technology Studies* 28, no. 3 (2015): 3–25; Paul Benneworth and Ben W. Jongbloed, "Who Matters to Universities? A Stakeholder Perspective on Humanities, Arts, and Social Sciences Valorization," *Higher Education* 59, no. 5 (2010): 567–588; Caragh Brosnan and Mike Michael, "Enacting the 'Neuro' in Practice: Translational Research, Adhesion and the Promise of Porosity," *Social Studies of Science* 44, no. 5 (2014): 680–700.

25. Maura Borrego and Lynita K. Newswander, "Definitions of Interdisciplinary Research: Toward Graduate-Level Interdisciplinary Learning Outcomes," *Review of Higher Education* 34, no. 1 (2010): 61–84.

26. In some recent studies of professionalization, for example, scholars have shown that the definition and institutionalization of the standardized concepts of "professionalism" and "professional identity" are embedded in specific social and cultural contexts—along academic, administrative, clinician, and specialty lines—that impose disparate visions of appropriate professional behavior. Frederic W. Hafferty and Brian Castellani, "The Increasing Complexities of Professionalism," *Academic Medicine* 85, no. 2 (2010): 288–301; Tania M. Jenkins, "Dual Autonomies, Divergent Approaches: How Stratification in Medical Education Shapes Approaches to Patient Care," *Journal of Health and Social Behavior* 59, no. 2 (2018): 268–282; Kellogg, *Challenging Operations*; Pål Erling Martinussen and Jon Magnussen, "Resisting Market-Inspired Reform in Healthcare: The Role of Professional Subcultures in Medicine," *Social Science and Medicine* 73, no. 2 (2011): 193–200; Daniel Menchik, "Interdependent Career Types and Divergent Standpoints on the Use of Advanced Technology in Medicine," *Journal of Health and Social Behavior* 58, no. 4 (2017): 488–502; stef m. shuster, *Trans Medicine: The Emergence and Practice of Treating Gender* (New York: New York University Press, 2021); LaTonya J. Trotter, "A Dream Deferred: Professional Projects as Racial Projects in US Medicine," in *The Routledge Handbook on the American Dream*, ed. Robert C. Hauhart and Mitja Sardoc (New York: Routledge, 2022), 331–351; Kelly Underman, *Feeling Medicine: How the Pelvic Exam Shapes Medical Training* (New York: New York University Press, 2020); Kelly Underman and Laura E. Hirshfield, "Detached Concern? Emotional Socialization in Twenty-First Century Medical Education," *Social Science and Medicine* 160, no. 1 (2016): 94–101; Adia Harvey Wingfield, *Flatlining: Race, Work, and Health Care in the New Economy* (Berkeley: University of California Press, 2019). For example, Kellogg, in *Challenging Operations*, showed how advocates of surgical interns'

hours reform were a diverse group of interns with marginalized or alternative social identities. This diverse group of women, other-specialty interns, men of color, and egalitarian men dedicated to their family were more likely to support hours reform precisely because their social identities were not valued in the traditional professional culture valorizing white "macho" men.

27. Critical race, postcolonial, and feminist scholars have drawn attention to how knowledge-producing and knowledge-applying institutions are steeped in white supremacy, imperialism, misogyny, heteronormativity, and their intersections. *Who* populated these institutions was just as important and inseparable from their epistemic limitations. Regarding the who, while historical practices made white cishet European men the privileged, this privilege lingered both through legacy and covert practices, as Glenn E. Bracey and Wendy Leo Moore wrote:

> White institutional space is created through a process that begins with whites excluding people of color . . . during a formative period in the history of an organization. During this period, whites populate all influential posts within the institution and create institutional logics—norms of operation, organizational structures, curricula, criteria for membership and leadership—which imbed white norms into the fabric of the institution's structure and culture. Although the norms are white, they are rarely marked as such. Consequently, racially biased institutional norms [appear] race neutral and merely characteristic of the institution . . . masking inherent institutional racism. Upon this tacitly racist foundation, institutional inertia and actors build a robust culture that privileges whites by vesting power in white leaders' hands, populating the organization with white membership, orienting activities toward serving and comforting whites and negatively sanctioning non-white norms.

Glenn E. Bracey and Wendy Leo Moore, "'Race Tests': Racial Boundary Maintenance in White Evangelical Churches," *Sociological Inquiry* 87, no. 2 (2017): 285. With this point of departure, the medical profession's epistemic limitations emerged around what knowledge was valued and what was not. As bell hooks has written, "emotional connections tend to be suspect in a world where the mind is valued above all else, where the idea that one should be and can be objective is paramount." bell hooks, *Teaching Community: A Pedagogy of Hope* (New York: Routledge, 2003), 127. Palmer Parker has similarly written how this stems from "the domineering mentality of objectivism . . . once the objectivist has 'the facts,' no listening is required, no other points of view are needed." Palmer Parker, *To Know as We Are Known: Education as a Spiritual Journey* (New York: HarperOne, 1983). And as Julian Go has argued further about the conflation of knowledge and knower: "The Cartesian Knower: 'he' who was rational, contemplative, and objective so he could transcend his immediate social location, observe from afar, and thus produce universal knowledge." Julian Go, "Race, Empire, and Epistemic Exclusion: Or the Structures of Sociological Thought," *Sociological Theory* 38, no. 2 (2020): 84. As an example, Go mentioned that W. E. B. Du Bois was not chosen to do the study of American race relations by Carnegie because there were "objectivity concerns" that he would be too biased because he was a Black man. And in showing that this inequity is still present, in their study of the professional culture in U.S. STEMM departments, Mary Blair-Loy and Erin Cech found that those who were not white or Asian men were less likely to be celebrated as geniuses and more likely to be seen as "diversity hires." Mary Blair-Loy and Erin Cech, *Misconceiving Merit: Paradoxes of Excellence and Devotion in Academic Science and Engineering* (Chicago: University of Chicago Press, 2022).

28. Critical curricular studies have pointed out how curricular practices are utilized to maintain the white supremacist and capitalistic status quo. Neo-Marxist scholars who critically evaluate how institutions of education operate depict schools "as agents of ideological control which function to reproduce and maintain dominant beliefs, values, and norms." Henry A. Giroux and Anthony N. Penna, "Social Education in the Classroom: The Dynamics of the Hidden Curriculum," *Theory and Research in Social Education* 7, no. 1 (1979): 26. In this approach, they point out that students learn social reproduction through classroom relationships and students learn false consciousness depending on what knowledge is taught, where in the institution's "failure lies in its inability to illuminate how social and political structures function to mask reality and promote ideological hegemony" (Giroux and Penna, p. 25). In their study of higher education and how students of color are treated, Eric Margolis and Mary Romero point out that curricular practices must be "seen as essential to the preserving of the existing social privilege, interests, and knowledge of one element of the population at the expense of less powerful groups. Most often this took the form of attempting to guarantee expert and scientific control in society, to eliminate or 'socialize' unwanted racial or ethnic groups or characteristics or to produce an economically efficient group of citizens." Eric Margolis and Mary Romero, "The Department Is Very Male,

Very White, Very Old, and Very Conservative: The Functioning of the Hidden Curriculum in Graduate Sociology Departments," *Harvard Educational Review* 68, no. 1 (1998): 34.

29. Because of the multiple purposes and meanings embedded in institutions of education, "polysemy makes universities extraordinarily flexible social mechanisms." Charlie Eaton and Mitchell L. Stevens, "Universities as Peculiar Organizations," *Sociology Compass* 14, no. 3 (2020): e12768.

30. As Dr. Carpano, a white male social scientist who had a joint appointment in his school of liberal arts and at his medical school, said to me about medical students: "They are the best of the best of the best and they are told that they are really great and ultimately will get automatic six-figure salaries and everyone worships them." Frederic W. Hafferty and Ronald Franks have written that "medical training at its root is a process of moral enculturation . . . transmitting normative rules regarding behavior and emotions." Frederic W. Hafferty and Ronald Franks, "The Hidden Curriculum, Ethics Teaching, and the Structure of Medical Education," *Academic Medicine* 69, no. 11 (1994): 861. Other medical sociologists have also depicted the moral socialization of medical students, whether it is the in-house monitoring of mistakes (Charles L. Bosk, *Forgive and Remember: Managing Medical Failure* [Chicago: University of Chicago Press, 1979])—and the subsequent "price of perfection" (Charles L. Bosk, *The Price of Perfection* [Baltimore, MD: Eastern Sociological Society, 2023])—or that the altruistic orientation allows the profession not to think of itself critically (Eliot Freidson, *Profession of Medicine: A Study of the Sociology of Applied Knowledge* [New York: Dodd, Mead, 1970]). Medicine, in its professionalized form in the United States, is white liberalism par excellence.

31. Alexandra H. Vinson, "'Constrained Collaboration': Patient Empowerment Discourse as Resource for Countervailing Power," *Sociology of Health and Illness* 38, no. 8 (2016): 1364–1378.

32. Anna Foster and Kathleen Kendall, "The Experience of Teaching Biomedical Science Subjects to UK Medical Students," [version 1; not peer reviewed], *MedEdPublish* 13 (2023): 61 (slides), https://doi.org/10.21955/mep.1115231.1.

33. LaTonya Trotter, keynote address at a preconference on the Social Transformation of the Sociology of Health Professions Education at the American Sociological Association annual meeting, August 17, 2023.

34. Historian John Hoberman has written about how "the physician's authority and autonomy can promote a socially conservative identity that resists both personal self-examination and social reforms" and that the medical profession has not confronted racism, both in its social distance, naivete, and "well

meaning . . . ritualized expressions of concern." John Hoberman, *Black and Blue: The Origins and Consequences of Medical Racism* (Berkeley: University of California Press, 2012), 9. This is in spite of the host of documented health and health-care inequalities, especially those patterned by race and racism: Ruha Benjamin, "Catching Our Breath: Critical Race STS and the Carceral Imagination," *Engaging Science, Technology, and Society* 2, no. 1 (2016): 145–156; Tony N. Brown, "Being Black and Feeling Blue: The Mental Health Consequences of Racial Discrimination," *Race and Society* 2, no. 2 (2000): 117–131; Phil Brown et al., "The Health Politics of Asthma: Environmental Justice and Collective Illness Experience in the United States," *Social Science and Medicine* 57, no. 3 (2003): 453–464; Ana V. Diez-Roux and Christina Mair, "Neighborhoods and Health," *Annals of the New York Academy of the Sciences* 1186, no. 1 (2010): 125–145; Bruce G. Link and Jo Phelan, "Social Conditions as Fundamental Causes of Disease," *Journal of Health and Social Behavior*, extra issue (1995): 80–94; David R. Williams, "Miles to Go Before We Sleep: Racial Inequalities in Health," *Journal of Health and Social Behavior* 53, no. 3 (2012): 279–295.

And the medical profession is part of the problem, whether one considers the provision of health care (Arthur L. Greil et al., "Race-Ethnicity and Medical Services for Infertility: Stratified Reproduction in a Population-Based Sample of U.S. Women," *Journal of Health and Social Behavior* 52, no. 4 [2011]: 493–509; Irena Stepanikova, "Racial-Ethnic Biases, Time Pressure, and Medical Decisions," *Journal of Health and Social Behavior* 53, no. 3 [2010]: 329–343; Michelle van Ryn and Steven S. Fu, "Paved with Good Intentions: Do Public Health and Human Service Providers Contribute to Racial/Ethnic Disparities in Health?," *American Journal of Public Health* 93, no. 2 [2003]: 248–255), practices of clinical research (Michael A. Byrd and Linda A. Clayton, "Race, Medicine and Healthcare in the United States: A Historical Survey," *Journal of the National Medical Association* 93, no. 3 [2001]: 11–34; Steven Epstein, *Inclusion: The Politics of Difference in Medical Research* [Chicago: University of Chicago Press, 2007]; Vanessa N. Gamble, "Under the Shadow of Tuskegee: African Americans and Healthcare," *American Journal of Public Health* 87, no. 11 [1997]: 1773–1778), or the composition of the profession itself (Joe R. Feagin and Zinobia Bennefield, "Systemic Racism and U.S. Healthcare," *Social Science and Medicine* 103, no. 1 [2014]: 7–14). The medical profession has historically disregarded or perpetuated racial inequalities in the United States. For more on how the medical profession trains its initiates, see Tania M. Jenkins et al., "The Resurgence of Medical Education in Sociology: A Return to Our Roots and an Agenda for the Future," *Journal of Health and Social Behavior* 62, no. 3 (2021): 255–270; Hoberman, *Black and Blue*.

35. Taking this moral framing seriously illuminated how or why curricular practices were seen as *the* solutions to bigger structural problems in the first place—medical educators failed to see how much their profession was part of the problem.

36. Helen Church and Megan Elizabeth Lincoln Brown, "Rise of the Med-Edists: Achieving a Critical Mass of Non-Practicing Clinicians Within Medical Education," *Medical Education* 56, no. 12 (2022): 1160–1163.

37. As Go asserts, the colonial world was a *source* of information for the colonizers; they were objects to be observed, not subjects with agency. They were raw data, not humans: "The claim was that, although nonwhite societies and peoples could not produce valid sociological knowledge, they could serve as analytic objects, providing data points for the (mostly evolutionary) social theories developed by white metropolitan sociologists." Go, "Race, Empire, and Epistemic Exclusion," 85. In professional medicine, "particularly those who view the knowledge base and application of science as value-neutral, 'objective', and therefore transcultural . . . they are not inclined to acknowledge the social and cultural matter" (Hafferty and Franks, "The Hidden Curriculum, Ethics Teaching, and the Structure of Medical Education," 863). In contrast, feminist, postcolonial, Indigenous approaches value perspective talking, collaboration, sharing credit, and humility.

    See also George Steinmetz, *The Politics of Method in the Human Sciences: Positivism and Its Epistemological Others* (Durham, NC: Duke University Press, 2005); Seth M. Holmes, Angela Jenks, and Scott Stonington, "Clinical Subjectivation: Anthropologies of Contemporary Biomedical Training," *Culture, Medicine, and Psychiatry* 35, no. 2 (2011): 105–112; Michelle Murphy, "Immodest Witnessing: The Epistemology of Vaginal Self-Examination in the U.S. Feminist Self-Help Movement," *Feminist Studies* 30, no. 1 (2004): 115–147.

38. Go, "Race, Empire, and Epistemic Exclusion."

39. Blair-Loy and Cech show how equity and inclusion work are viewed as "too political" in STEMM fields. Blair-Loy and Erin Cech, *Misconceiving Merit*.

40. Mary Blair-Loy, *Competing Devotions: Career and Family Among Women Executives* (Cambridge, MA: Harvard University Press, 2005); Tressie McMillan Cottom, *Thick: And Other Essays* (New York: The New Press, 2018).

41. This terminology stems from the remarks of former president of the American Psychiatric Association, Steven Sharfstein. In his presidential address, he

was reflecting on the profession's swing to solely biomedical models, stating: "We must examine the fact that as a profession, we have allowed the biopsychosocial model to become the bio-bio-bio model." Steven S. Sharfstein, "Big Pharma and American Psychiatry: The Good, the Bad, and the Ugly," *Psychiatric News* (2005), https://doi.org/10.1176/pn.40.16.00400003.

42. Deborah Gordon, "Clinical Science and Clinical Expertise: Changing Boundaries Between Art and Science in Medicine," in *Biomedicine Examined*, ed. Margaret Lock and Deborah Gordon (Amsterdam: Kluwer-Academic, 1988), 257–295.

43. Kenneth M. Ludmerer, *Learning to Heal: The Development of American Medical Education* (New York: Basic Books, 1985); Kenneth M. Ludmerer, *Time to Heal: American Medical Education from the Turn of the Century to the Era of Managed Care* (New York: Oxford University Press, 1999); William C. McGaghie, "Assessing Readiness for Medical Education: Evolution of the Medical College Admission Test," *Journal of the American Medical Association* 288, no. 9 (2002): 1085–1090.

44. I am grateful for a conversation with Alexandra Vinson for this formulation.

45. "Case oriented methods traditionally have framed the domain of ethics almost entirely within the patient-provider relationship . . . what becomes lost is a view of how medicine in general or medical schools in particular might be considered as moral agents or moral entities." Hafferty and Franks, "The Hidden Curriculum, Ethics Teaching, and the Structure of Medical Education," 864. See also Seth M. Holmes and Maya Pointe, "En-case-ing the Patient: Disciplining Uncertainty in Medical Student Patient Presentations," *Culture Medicine and Psychiatry* 35, no. 1 (2013): 163–182.

46. Seamster and Ray, "Against Teleology in the Study of Race," 316. This progress paradigm can be seen in how the medical profession understands its relationship to racial progress. Biological racial classifications—from Linnaeus's 1785 taxonomy to physiognomy, anthropometry, phrenology, ethnology, eugenics, retroactively described as pseudoscience when, in fact, it was scientific racism, which Seamster and Ray describe as an action of "sanitizing white violence"— yielded a "biological separation (by species)" that then was followed by one of "cultural separation (by time)" (320). And *interest convergence* "explains progression and retrenchment" in that "multiculturalism, diversity, and inclusion have been appropriated and rearticulated in educational and corporate settings in ways that retrench and solidify white institutional space." Jennifer C. Mueller, "Racial Ideology or Racial Ignorance? An Alternative Theory of Racial Cognition," *Sociological Theory* 38, no. 2 (2020): 156; Derrick A. Bell

Jr., "Brown v. Board of Education and the Interest-Convergence Dilemma," *Harvard Law Review* 93, no. 3 (1980): 518–533.

47. George Lipsitz, "The Possessive Investment in Whiteness: Racialized Social Democracy and the 'White' Problem in American Studies," *American Quarterly* 47, no. 3 (1995): 369–387. As Mueller writes, "people in power often have the unique capacity and incentive to suppress knowledge and nurture ignorance, not just interpersonally but also by using institutions to structure broad architectures of nonknowledge" ("Racial Ideology or Racial Ignorance?," 145). Look no further than the *Journal of the American Medical Association* (JAMA)'s podcast. In a since-deleted episode, entitled "Structural Racism for Doctors—What Is It?," the white host and guest claimed not only ignorance about the subject but also even skepticism about it, undermining the significance of structural racism for their audience in early 2021. Clarence C. Gravlee, "How Whiteness Works: JAMA and the Refusals of White Supremacy," *Somatosphere*, March 27, 2021, https://somatosphere.com/2021/how-whiteness-works.html/; Mueller, "Racial Ideology or Racial Ignorance?," 142–169.

48. While medical school faculty of color have written autobiographically about their experiences, medical sociology as a subfield has very little empirical data on how racial minorities may be disproportionately affected during their professional training. Kali D. Cyrus, "Medical Education and the Minority Tax," *Journal of the American Medical Association* 317, no. 18 (2017): 1833–1834; Damon Tweedy, *Black Man in a White Coat* (New York: Picador, 2015). In one of the few studies of race and medical students, a prospective observational study of 3,547 students from a random stratified sample of forty-nine U.S. medical schools asked students about their implicit racial biases. Michelle van Ryn et al., "Medical School Experiences Associated with Change in Implicit Racial Bias Among 3547 Students: A Medical Student CHANGES Study Report," *Journal of General Internal Medicine* 30, no. 12 (2015): 1754. Michelle van Ryn et al. conclude that instructors often do not exhibit "sufficient depth of knowledge" when teaching the didactic material on race and that interracial contact impacts students' implicit racial attitudes. This latter finding about interracial contact posits that white students who reported "favorable" contact with students and faculty of color were more likely to have fewer implicit racial biases toward people of color. While van Ryn et al.'s study is important for considering racial bias in medical training, the scholars do not explore the interactions that constitute "favorable contact" to identify the process by which these biases may be lessened, nor do the scholars consider the experiences of students of color.

That said, sociological research on underrepresented minority students in other white-dominated institutions of education has shown that "numerical rarity by race significantly increases 'token stress.'" Pamela Brayboy Jackson, Peggy Thoits, and Howard F. Taylor, "Composition of the Workplace and Psychological Well-Being: The Effects of Tokenism on America's Black Elite," *Social Forces* 74, no. 2 (1995): 543. Studies of graduate students of color in STEMM fields indicate that underrepresented students experience greater isolation, discrimination, microaggressions, mental health issues, and mentoring gaps. Maria Ong et al., "Inside the Double Bind: A Synthesis of Empirical Research on Undergraduate and Graduate Women of Color in Science, Technology, Engineering, and Mathematics," *Harvard Educational Review* 81, no. 2 (2011): 172–209; Lucas Torres, Mark W. Driscoll, and Anthony L. Burrow, "Racial Microaggressions and Psychological Functioning Among Highly Achieving African-Americans: A Mixed-Methods Approach," *Journal of Social and Clinical Psychology* 29, no. 10 (2010): 1074–1099. Scholars have also shown that graduate students of color pursuing academic careers face assumptions about their criminality, intellectual worth, and belonging. David L. Brunsma, David G. Embrick, and Jean H. Shin, "Graduate Students of Color: Race, Racism, and Mentoring in the White Waters of Academia," *Sociology of Race and Ethnicity* 3, no. 1 (2017): 1–13.

49. Elan Burton et al., "Assessment of Bias in Patient Safety Reporting Systems Categorized by Physician Gender, Race and Ethnicity, and Faculty Rank," *Journal of the American Medical Association Network Open* 5, no. 5 (2022): e2213234.

50. For work on learning about race and impact on health care, see Brooke A. Cunningham et al., "Physicians' Anxiety Due to Uncertainty and Use of Race in Medical Decision Making," *Medical Care* 52, no. 8 (2014): 728–733; Michelle van Ryn et al., "The Impact of Racism on Clinician Cognition, Behavior, and Clinical Decision Making," *DuBois Review* 8, no. 1 (2011): 199–218. For trans and gender minority health care, see Ning Hsieh and stef. m. shuster, "Health and Health Care of Sexual and Gender Minorities," *Journal of Health and Social Behavior* 62, no. 2 (2021): 318–333; shuster, *Trans Medicine*.

51. Jonathan Kahn, "Pills for Prejudice: Implicit Bias and Technical Fix for Racism," *American Journal of Law and Medicine* 43 (2017): 263–278; Jamie L. Manzer and Ann V. Bell, "We're a Little Biased: Medicine and the Management of Bias Through the Case of Contraception," *Journal of Health and Social Behavior* 62, no. 2 (2021): 120–135.

52. Michael W. Rabow et al., "Insisting on the Healer's Art: The Implications of Required Participation in a Medical School Course on Values and

Humanism," *Teaching and Learning in Medicine* 28, no. 1 (2016): 61–71; Helen Riess and Liz Neporent, *The Empathy Effect: Seven Neuroscience-Based Keys for Transforming the Way We Live, Love, Work, and Connect Across Differences* (Boston: Sounds True Publishing, 2018); Stephen Tzreciak and Anthony Mazzarelli, *Compassionomics: The Revolutionary Scientific Evidence That Caring Makes a Difference* (New York: Studer, 2019).

53. Elle Lett et al., "Health Equity Tourism: Ravaging the Justice Landscape," *Journal of Medical Systems* 46, no. 17 (2022): 2.

54. Lett et al., "Health Equity Tourism," 2.

55. Alexandra H. Vinson, "Teaching the Work of Doctoring: How the Medical Profession Adapts to Change" (PhD diss., University of California San Diego, 2015).

56. Sara Ahmed, *Complaint!* (Durham, NC: Duke University Press, 2021).

57. Michel Antelby, *Manufacturing Morals: The Values of Silence in Business School Education* (Chicago: University of Chicago Press, 2013); Wendy Leo Moore, *Reproducing Racism: White Space, Elite Law Schools, and Racial Inequality* (New York: Rowman and Littlefield, 2008); Michael Sierra-Arevalo, *The Danger Imperative: Violence, Death, and the Soul of Policing* (New York: Columbia University Press, 2024).

58. Ann Morning, *The Nature of Race: How Scientists Think and Teach About Human Difference* (Berkeley: University of California Press, 2011); Aviad Raz and Judith Fadlon, "'We Came to Talk with the People Behind the Disease': Communication and Control in Medical Education," *Culture, Medicine and Psychiatry* 30, no. 1 (2006): 55–75; Janet K. Shim, *Heart-Sick: The Politics of Risk, Inequality, and Heart Disease* (New York: New York University Press, 2014).

1. CURRICULAR PRACTICES AND PROFESSIONAL POWER

1. Carlyle Jacobsen, "Student Selection Problems: ROUND TABLE A," *Journal of Medical Education* 25, no. 1 (1950): 8.

2. As the president of Harvard at the time, James B. Conant, stated in 1939, "[M]any deans, professors, and members of the medical profession protest that what they all desire is a man with a liberal education, not a man with four years loaded with the premedical sciences." As cited in Kenneth M. Ludmerer, *Learning to Heal: The Development of American Medical Education* (New York: Basic Books, 1985), 277.

3. Association of American Medical Colleges, "Diversity in Medical Education: Facts and Figures 2016," Vol. 6, *Facts and Figures Report* (Washington, DC: AAMC, 2016); Jerome Karabel, *The Chosen: The Hidden History of Admission and Exclusion at Harvard, Yale, and Princeton* (New York: Houghton Mifflin, 2005); Shamus R. Khan, *Privilege: The Making of an Adolescent Elite at St. Paul's School* (Princeton, NJ: Princeton University Press, 2011); Natasha K. Warikoo, *The Diversity Bargain: And Other Dilemmas of Race, Admissions, and Meritocracy at Elite Universities* (Chicago: University of Chicago Press, 2016).

4. Association of American Medical Colleges, "Total Enrollment by U.S. Medical School and Race/Ethnicity, 2017–2018," vol. 3, *FACTS: Applicants, Matriculants, Enrollment, Graduates, MD-PhD, and Residency Applicants Data* (Washington, DC: AAMC, 2018).

5. Stacy J. Williams, Laura Pecenco, and Mary Blair-Loy, "Medical Professions: The Status of Women and Men" (La Jolla, CA: University of California San Diego, 2013).

6. Oscar E. Dimant, Tiffany E. Cook, Richard E. Green, and Asa E. Radix, "Experiences of Transgender and Gender Nonbinary Medical Students and Physicians," *Transgender Health* 4, no. 1 (2019): 209–216; Josef Madrigal, Sarah Rudasil, Zachary Tran, Jonathan Bergman, and Peyman Benharash, "Sexual and Gender Minority Identity in Undergraduate Medical Education: Impact on Experience and Career Trajectory," *PLoS One* 16, no. 11 (2021): e0260387; Jules L. Madzia, "Inequality in Medical Professionalization and Specialization" (PhD diss., University of Cincinnati, 2023).

7. Association of American Medical Colleges, "Total Enrollment by U.S. Medical School." Only 11 percent of medical school deans in 2019 were from underrepresented racial backgrounds. Autumn Nobles et al., "Stalled Progress: Medical School Dean Demographics," *Journal of the American Board of Family Medicine* 35, no. 1 (2022): 163–168.

8. Association of American Medical Colleges, *U.S. Medical School Deans by Dean Type and Race/Ethnicity* (Washington, DC: AAMC), 2023. Asian Americans hold 20 percent of clinical faculty positions but half of that in chair positions, and between 1997 and 2008, there were no Asian American deans. Peter T. Yu et al., "Minorities Struggle to Advance in Academic Medicine: A 12-Year Review of Diversity at the Highest Levels of America's Teaching Institutions," *Journal of Surgical Residency* 182, no. 2 (2013): 212–218.

9. Association of American Medical Colleges, "Matriculating Student Questionnaire" (Washington, DC: AAMC, 2016).

10. Mytien Nguyen, Mayur M. Desai, and Tonya L. Fancher, "Temporal Trends in Childhood Household Income Among Applicants and Matriculants to Medical School and the Likelihood of Acceptance by Income, 2014–2019," *Journal of the American Medical Association* (2023), doi:10.1001/jama.2023.5654; David E. Velasquez, Arman A. Shahriar, and Fidencio Saldana, "Economic Disparity and the Physician Pipeline—Medicine's Uphill Battle." *Journal of General Internal Medicine* (2023), doi:10.1007/s11606-023-08109-3.

11. Magali S. Larson, "Professionalism: Rise and Fall," *International Journal of Health Services* 9, no. 4 (1979): 607–627.

12. Because of the limits of biomedical knowledge and skill, physicians' work centered on palliative care and home visits; because of the cultural values of the U.S. population, patients were more self-reliant and skeptical of science. Paul Starr, *The Social Transformation of American Medicine* (New York: Basic Books, 1982).

13. In fact, as Francis Scott Smyth, a leader in the medical profession, described in 1962, "the success of great physicians in the past has often rested as much on the psychosocial base as a biophysical one. Much of the former was intuitive. Indeed, it has been hinted that the treatment of patients as persons and members of society compensated for the inadequacy of their biophysical knowledge." Francis Scott Smyth, "The Place of the Humanities and Social Sciences in the Education of Physicians," *Journal of Medical Education* 37, no. 5 (1962): 496.

14. Ludmerer, *Learning to Heal*; Starr, *The Social Transformation of American Medicine*.

15. Moya Bailey, "The Flexner Report: Standardizing Medical Students Through Region-, Gender-, and Race-Based Hierarchies," *American Journal of Law and Medicine* 43 (2017): 209–223; Rana Hogarth, *Medicalizing Blackness: Making Racial Difference in the Atlantic World, 1780–1840* (Raleigh: University of North Carolina Press, 2017); Deidre Cooper Owens, *Medical Bondage: Race, Gender, and the Origins of American Gynecology* (Athens: University of Georgia Press, 2017); LaTonya J. Trotter, "A Dream Deferred: Professional Projects as Racial Projects in US Medicine," in *The Routledge Handbook on the American Dream*, ed. Robert C. Hauhart and Mitja Sardoc (New York: Routledge, 2022), 331–351; Christopher Willoughby, *Masters of Health: Racial Sciences and Slavery in U.S. Medical Schools* (Raleigh: University of North Carolina Press, 2022).

16. Ludmerer, *Learning to Heal*; Abraham Flexner, *Medical Education in the United States and Canada: A Report to the Carnegie Foundation for the Advancement of Teaching*, Bulletin Number Four (New York: The Carnegie Foundation, 1910).

17. This is in line with many theories of professions (e.g., Eliot Freidson, *Profession of Medicine: A Study of the Sociology of Applied Knowledge* [New York: Dodd, Mead, 1970]; Andrew Abbott, *The Systems of the Professions: An Essay on the Division of Expert Labor* [Chicago: University of Chicago Press, 1988]).

18. Victor Ray, "A Theory of Racialized Organizations," *American Sociological Review* 84, no. 1 (2019): 26–53.

19. While the idealized physician was indeed a "scientific practitioner," as Flexner (*Medical Education in the United States and Canada*, 26) wrote, science in and of itself was inadequate for the training of future professionals; physicians also needed "insight and sympathy" and the knowledge that, "directly or indirectly, disease has been found to depend largely on unpropitious environments . . . the physician's function is fast becoming social and preventative, rather than individual and curative."

20. David B. Tyler, "A University Is an Institution That Has Trouble with Its Medical School," *Journal of Medical Education* 35, no. 8 (1960): 792.

21. Ludmerer, *Learning to Heal*, 115.

22. Trotter, "A Dream Deferred."

23. Bailey, "The Flexner Report."

24. Warren Weaver, "Medicine: The New Science and the Old Art," *Journal of Medical Education* 35, no. 4 (1960): 314.

25. Wilder Penfield, "Medical School Admissions," *Journal of the Association of American Medical Colleges* 33, no. 7 (1958): 854; Melvin A. Casberg, "Medical Education Takes Inventory," *Journal of the Association of American Medical Colleges* 25, no. 5 (1950): 306; William E. Cadbury Jr., Charles Dawson, Thomas Hunter, and Richard Masland, "The Responsibility of the Arts College to the Student Planning the Study of Medicine," *Journal of the Association of American Medical Colleges* 26, no. 3 (1951): 170; Robert Collier Page, "The Doctor for Tomorrow's Needs," *Journal of the Association of American Medical Colleges* 27, no. 2 (1952): 91.

26. Created in 1928, the MCAT underwent six substantial revisions between then and 2015. For a history of the MCAT in the twentieth century, see William C. McGaghie, "Assessing Readiness for Medical Education: Evolution of the Medical College Admission Test," *Journal of the American Medical Association* 288, no. 9 (2002): 1085–1090.

27. William W. Stiles, Francis Scott Smyth, and Mathea Reuter, "Individual and Community Health Instruction in the Premedical Curriculum," *Journal of Medical Education* 28, no. 6 (1953): 29.

28. Rex F. Arragon, "Humanities and Medical Education," *Journal of Medical Education* 35, no. 10 (1960): 908.

29. Henry Sigerist, "Medical History in the Medical Schools of the United States," *Bulletin of the History of Medicine* 7, no. 6 (1939): 627–662.

30. Otto E. Guttentag, "A Course Entitled 'The Medical Attitude': An Orientation in the Foundations of Medical Thought," *Journal of Medical Education* 35, no. 10 (1960): 903.

31. Karabel, *The Chosen*.

32. Lauren A. Rivera, *Pedigree: How Elite Students Get Elite Jobs* (Princeton, NJ: Princeton University Press, 2015). In Rivera's account of how employers contribute to elite reproduction, she found that socioeconomic sorting in hiring processes occurred through the use and interpretation of various signals. Employers were invested in looking for signals that potential hires were similar to them, in a process she calls *looking glass merit*. Employers "wanted new hires who 'fit' culturally and socially" with how current employees envisioned themselves (pp. 94, 112). She found that employers had an attendant belief that "being well-rounded could potentially reduce the risk of burnout or attrition" (p. 96). Following Bourdieu, Rivera noted that the curriculum vitae (CV) was essentially "institutionalized cultural capital" and thus line items that might require more time or money denoted the CV holder's "distance from necessity" (p. 110). Scholars elsewhere have documented how these extracurricular activities are classed. See, for example, Mitchell L. Stevens, *Creating a Class: College Admissions and the Education of Elites* (Cambridge, MA: Harvard University Press, 2007).

33. Starr, *The Social Transformation of American Medicine*. Once the physicians attained power, it did not take long for countervailing forces to check that power. To combat the consequences of the physicians' share of market power, other stakeholders entered the health-care system beginning in the 1960s, whether to defray rising costs (e.g., insurance companies, hospital administration) or to advocate on behalf of patients (e.g., bioethicists, Medicaid/Medicare, consumerism), culminating in a curtailing of the power and paternalism that many physicians held. By the 1970s, the medical profession began losing its dominance because it was subject to more standards, surveillance, patient consumerism, ethical guidelines, and democratization. Donald W. Light, "Introduction: Ironies of Success: A New History of the American Health Care 'System,'" *Journal of Health and Social Behavior* 45, no. 1 (2004): 1–24; John B. McKinlay and Lisa Marceau, "The End of the Golden Age of Doctoring," in *The Sociology of Health and Illness: Critical Perspectives*, 7th ed., ed. Rose Weitz (New York: Worth Publishers, 2002), 189–214.

34. Julian Go, "Race, Empire, and Epistemic Exclusion: Or the Structures of Sociological Thought," *Sociological Theory* 38, no. 2 (2020).

35. Ludmerer notes that, as medical schools expanded in the latter half of the twentieth century, medical students became their "forgotten members." Kenneth M. Ludmerer, *Time to Heal: American Medical Education from the Turn of the Century to the Era of Managed Care* (New York: Oxford University Press, 1999), 176.

36. Ludmerer, *Time to Heal*, 54.

37. Buttressed by the increased economization of scientific knowledge production, the body of knowledge undergirding the physical, engineering, and biological sciences grew, which in turn increased the number of higher education institutions and accredited medical schools and entrenched the federal government's support of biomedical research. Adele E. Clarke et al., "Biomedicalization: Technoscientific Transformations of Health, Illness, and U.S. Biomedicine," *American Sociological Review* 68, no. 2 (2003): 161–194; Renee Fox, "Training for Uncertainty," in *The Student-Physician: Introductory Studies in the Sociology of Medical Education*, ed. Robert K. Merton, George G. Reader, and Patricia L. Kendall (Cambridge, MA: Harvard University Press, 1957), 207–241.

38. McGaghie, "Assessing Readiness for Medical Education."

39. What constitutes medical humanities now is quite broad, as Brian Dolan explains: "When pressed to define 'medical humanities', it appears more inclusive than exclusive, thereby resisting conventional disciplinary identity. History of medicine, bioethics, narrative medicine, medicine in literature, creative writing, and various social sciences (for example, medical anthropology and sociology) are aspects of medical humanities programmes. However, it also embraces the creative arts, so that music, painting, reader's theatre, and dance are considered expressive of medical humanities. Anything that touches on the 'human condition,' 'the humanizing process,' or 'the humanist philosophy' becomes relevant." Brian Dolan, "History, Medical Humanities, and Medical Education," *Social History of Medicine* 23, no. 2 (2010): 394. That said, medical humanities—as a body of potential curricular practices—is not monolithic. Some critics have been critical of the focus on medicine, advocating that it be termed *health humanities* to be more inclusive. Howard Brody, "Defining the Medical Humanities: Three Conceptions and Three Narratives," *Journal of Medical Humanities* 32 (2011): 1–7. Still others are critical of some of its application—whether about what is taught as well as who is charged with the instruction. Some feel that it is a perversion of medical humanities' role and

purpose in medical education. Delese Wear, J. Zarconi, Arno Kumagai, and K. Cole-Kelly, "Slow Medical Education," *Academic Medicine* 90, no. 3 (2015): 289–293. Others describe a tension between who should be in charge of medical humanities education in medical schools—those with professional disciplinary training in a humanistic or social scientific field versus those "sensitive and thoughtful people who care passionately about medical education" yet do not "know a lot about philosophy or literature." Jack Coulehan, "What Is Medical Humanities and Why," *Lit Med Magazine* (2008): 1. In fact, a second wave of medical humanities has emerged in the United Kingdom in reaction to what they refer to as medical humanities "lite," which "rarely progressed beyond tinkering around the edges of medical education." Alan Bleakley, "Introduction: The Medical Humanities: A Mixed Weather Front on a Global Scale," in *Routledge Handbook of the Medical Humanities*, ed. Alan Bleakley (New York: Routledge, 2019): 1–28; Jane MacNaughton, "Medical Humanities' Challenge to Medicine," *Journal of Evaluation in Clinical Practice* 17 (2011): 927–932; Anne Whitehead and Angela Woods, *The Edinburgh Companion to the Critical Medical Humanities* (Edinburgh: Edinburgh University Press, 2016).

40. Medical humanities, in the form of bioethics, became embedded in the institutional fabric of American medical schools. Edmund Pellegrino, "Medical History and Medical Education: Points of Engagement." *Clio Medica* 10, no. 3 (1975): 295–303; Edmund Pellegrino, "The Virtuous Physician and the Ethics of Medicine," in *Virtue and Medicine: Explorations in the Character of Medicine*, ed. Earl E. Shelp (Dordrecht: Reidel, 1985), 237–255.

41. As an example of a "thick" use of the humanities that was abandoned (see, for example, John H. Evans, *Playing God? Human Genetic Engineering and the Rationalization of Public Bioethical Debate* [Chicago: University of Chicago Press, 2002]), take the description provided by Edmund Pellegrino, a central figure in the rise of bioethics, who described the agenda for a "humanities in medicine" and drew on the legacy of medical history in medical education: "The engagement of medical history with medical education is itself a model of the way humanities in general might be more effective in the university and in society . . . consistent with the traditional aim of the liberal arts—to liberate the mind from subservience to the ideas of others." Pellegrino, "Medical History and Medical Education," 301. See also Dolan, "History, Medical Humanities, and Medical Education"; H. Tristram Engelhardt, "Managed Care and the Deprofessionalization of Medicine," in *The Ethics of Managed Care: Professional Integrity and Patient Rights*, ed. W. B.

Bondeson and J. W. Jones (Amsterdam: Kluwer, 2001), 93–108; Marie R. Haug, "A Re-examination of the Hypothesis of Physician Deprofessionalization," *Milbank Memorial Fund Quarterly* 66, no. 2 (1988): 48–56; Mary E. Kollmer Horton, "A (Un)Natural Alliance: Medical Education and the Humanities," (PhD diss., Emory University, 2020).

42. Dolan, "History, Medical Humanities, and Medical Education."

43. Academia has evolved over the course of the twentieth century, too. Scholars from a variety of disciplines have written extensively about the crisis of the liberal arts in a market-driven era. Burton R. Clark, *The Higher Education System: Academic Organization in Cross-National Perspective* (Berkeley: University of California Press, 1983); Frank Donoghue, *The Last Professors: The Corporate University and the Fate of the Humanities* (New York: Fordham University Press, 2008); Louis Menand, *The Marketplace of Ideas: Reform and Resistance in the American University* (New York: Norton, 2010). Leaders of institutions of higher education respond to market, student, and public pressures to become more economized and applied to emphasize revenue generation, productive returns from research, and increasing the earnings of their graduates. Ami Zusman, "Challenges Facing Higher Education in the Twenty-First Century," in *American Higher Education in the Twenty-First Century*, ed. Philip G. Altbach, Robert O. Berdahl, and Patricia J. Gumport (Baltimore, MD: Johns Hopkins University Press, 2005), 115–160. Scholars argue that this trend means that the traditional liberal arts' majors, curricula, and departments are in peril. Martin Trow, "The Campus as a Context for Learning," in *Twentieth-Century Higher Education: Elite to Mass to Universal*, ed. Michael Burrage (Baltimore, MD: Johns Hopkins University Press, 2010), 303–318. Faculty members in humanities and social science disciplines have experienced declines in the number of majors they obtain (Steven Brint, *The Future of the City of Intellect: The Changing American University* [Palo Alto, CA: Stanford University Press, 2002]), the required amount of time students spend in their courses (Richard Arum and Josipa Roksa, *Academically Adrift: Limited Learning on College Campuses* [Chicago: University of Chicago Press, 2011]), and the funding of their departments and research (Tamar Lewin, "As Interest Fades in the Humanities, Colleges Worry," *New York Times* [October 30, 2013]). As the leadership and students within institutions of higher education devalued the liberal arts, they prioritized the "practical arts," or occupation-based fields of study such as nursing, business, or marketing (Steven Brint, Mark Riddle, Lori Turk-Bicakci, and Charles S. Levy, "From the Liberal to the Practical Arts in American Colleges and Universities: Organizational Analysis and

Curricular Change," *The Journal of Higher Education* 76, no. 2 [2005], 151–152).
In addition, academics in the biomedical, computer, and engineering sciences have "dramatically increased the[ir] wealth and authority . . . relative to th[ose] in the social sciences and the humanities" (Mitchell L. Stevens, Elizabeth Armstrong, and Richard Arum, "Sieve, Incubator, Temple, Hub: Empirical and Conceptual Advances in the Sociology of Higher Education," *Annual Review of Sociology* 34 [2008]: 138).

44. Eric Touya de Marienne, *The Case for the Humanities: Pedagogy, Polity, and Interdisciplinarity* (Baltimore, MD: Rowman and Littlefield, 2016), 2.

45. William R. Willard, "New Medical Schools: Some Preliminary Considerations," *Journal of Medical Education* 35, no. 2 (1960): 95–107. Historian Brian Dolan suggests that medical anthropology and the social and behavioral sciences replaced medical history from the ranks of medical education by the late 1970s. According to Chester Burns, a physician and medical historian, "just as social sciences had undermined the eminence of historical studies in collegiate education, they began to do the same for medical history in medical education after 1950." Chester Burns, "History in Medical Education: The Development of Current Trends in the United States," *Bulletin of the New York Academy of Medicine* 51, no. 7 (1975): 859. As both Donald W. Light ("Introduction: Strengthening Ties Between Specialties and Disciplines," *American Journal of Sociology* 97, no. 4 [1992]: 909–918) and Samuel W. Bloom (*The Word as Scalpel: History of Medical Sociology* [Oxford: Oxford University Press, 2002]) detail, it was no accident that medical sociology and medical anthropology in medical education were born out of social scientific alliances with psychiatry. The inclusion of psychiatry into general medical education and the increased funding of social scientific research and teaching by the National Institute of Mental Health jump-started the behavioral health movement in the 1960s. The medical profession found the social scientific and psychiatric insights into psychosocial components of human behavior to contribute to the strengthening of the doctor-patient relationship, or the "human relations side of medicine." Samuel W. Bloom, "The Role of the Sociologist in Medical Education," *Journal of Medical Education* 34, no. 7 (1959): 667; David Mechanic, "The Role of Sociology in Health Affairs," *Health Affairs* 9, no. 1 (1990): 85–97.

46. As Francis Scott Smyth described, "The education of the physician for the present and the future must provide a scientific and systematic acquaintance with both the sociological and the biological fields and methods for utilizing, for applying the principles in both. Physical factors involved in illness

are fundamental, but comprehensive medical care must include whatever the humanities and social sciences can contribute" (Smyth, "The Place of the Humanities and Social Sciences," 496).

47. National Institute of Child Health and Human Development, "Behavioral Sciences and Medical Education: A Report of Four Conferences" (Washington, DC: U.S. Department of Health, Education, and Welfare. Public Health Service, National Institutes of Health, 1970), DHEW Publication No. (NIH) 72–41.

48. John Romano, "Community Needs: The Student, the Medical School as It Exists Today," *Journal of Medical Education* 27, no. 3 (1952): 168; Cynthia R. Whitehead, Brian D. Hodges, and Zubin Austin, "Captive on a Carousel: Discourses of 'New' in Medical Education 1910–2010," *Advances in Health Sciences Education* 18 (2013): 755–768.

49. Alondra Nelson, *Body and Soul: The Black Panther Party and the Fight Against Medical Discrimination* (Minneapolis: University of Minnesota Press, 2011); Kelly Underman, *Feeling Medicine: How the Pelvic Exam Shapes Medical Training* (New York: New York University Press, 2020).

50. Lily M. Hoffman and Fitzhugh Mullan describe in detail a small group of medical student activists who were involved in the civil rights movement. Lily M. Hoffman, *The Politics of Knowledge: Activist Movements in Medicine and Planning* (Albany, NY: SUNY Press, 1989); Fitzhugh Mullan, *White Coat, Clenched Fist: The Political Education of an American Physician* (Ann Arbor: University of Michigan Press, 1976, 2006). At the time of his writing, Mullan was optimistic about change; decades later in his new preface he was outraged and dismayed: "The intersection between radical politics and American medicine does not occupy a large space" (Mullan, *White Coat, Clenched Fist*, ix). In his 1976 memoir, he documents the conservative and individualistic politics of the medical profession.

51. Tania M. Jenkins and Shalini Reddy, "Revisiting the Rationing of Medical Degrees in the United States," *Contexts* 15, no. 4 (2016): 36–41; Michael W. Byrd and Linda A. Clayton, eds., *Race, Medicine, and Healthcare in the U.S.* vol. 2 of *An American Health Dilemma* (New York: Routledge, 2002).

52. Cynthia R. Whitehead, Brian D. Hodges, and Zubin Austin, "Dissecting the Doctor: From Character to Characteristics in North American Medical Education," *Advances in Health Sciences Education* 18 (2013): 687–699.

53. Ruha Benjamin, "Cultura Obscura: Race, Power, and 'Culture Talk' in the Health Sciences." *American Journal of Law and Medicine* 43 (2017): 225–238; Khiara M. Bridges, *Reproducing Race: An Ethnography of Pregnancy as a Site of*

Racialization (Berkeley: University of California Press, 2011); Ray, "A Theory of Racialized Organizations."

54. Health disparities research is a broad field that examines why specific marginalized groups or a marginalized population have worse morbidity and mortality rates than the dominant group. In the United States, the federal government has many offices dedicated to the reduction and elimination of racial and ethnic disparities in health and health care. Six central bureaucratic bodies in the U.S. Department of Health and Human Services oversee the research and responses to these racial and ethnic disparities: National Institutes of Health's National Institute of Minority Health Disparities (NIMHD), the Agency for Health Research and Quality (AHRQ), the Health Resources and Services Administration's Office of Health Equity (HRSA-OHE) and Office for Minority Health (HRSA-OMH), Substance Abuse and Mental Health Services Administration (SAMHSA), the National Academies' Institute of Medicine (IOM), and the Centers for Disease Control and Prevention's Racial and Ethnic Approaches to Community Health (CDC-REACH). Under each of these bodies are hundreds of centers, institutes, hospitals, nonprofits, and for-profit consulting organizations that receive federal funding to conduct research and identify solutions to racial and ethnic disparities in health and health care.

55. B. D. Smedley, A. Y. Stith, A. R. Nelson, and Institute of Medicine (U.S.) Committee on Understanding and Eliminating Racial and Ethnic Disparities in Health Care, *Unequal Treatment: Confronting Racial and Ethnic Disparities in Health Care* (Washington, DC: National Academy Press, 2003).

56. This act created the National Center on Minority Health and Health Disparities within the National Institutes of Health (NIH) to "conduct and support research, training, dissemination of information, and other programs with respect to minority health conditions and other populations with health disparities" (S. 1880: sec. 101). Most important for medical education, however, was Title IV of the act (S. 1880: sec. 401, 402, 403), which outlined curricular initiatives. Following this act, the U.S. Department of Health and Human Services Office of Minority Health (HHS-OMH) created the National Standards on Culturally and Linguistically Appropriate Services (CLAS) in 2001. In 2002, the Health Resources and Services Administration (HRSA) established and funded the National Center for Cultural Competence, which oversaw planning and implementation recommendations for nationwide cultural competence measures. Additional acts at the federal level have institutionalized the goal of eliminating racial and ethnic disparities in health:

the Minority Health and Health Disparity Elimination Act of 2007 (S.1576), the Minority Health Improvement and Health Disparity Elimination Act (HR3333), and the Health Equity and Accountability Act (HR3014).

57. Cultural competence was defined by the Association of American Medical Colleges as a "set of congruent behaviors, knowledge, attitudes, and policies that come together in a system, organization, or among professionals that enables effective work in cross-cultural situations. 'Culture' refers to integrated patterns of human behavior that include the language, thoughts, actions, customs, beliefs, and institutions of racial, ethnic, social, or religious groups. 'Competence' implies having the capacity to function effectively as an individual or an organization within the context of the cultural beliefs, practices, and needs presented by patients and their communities." Association of American Medical Colleges, "Cultural Competence Education for Medical Students," (Washington, DC: AAMC, 2005). See also Arthur Kleinman, *Patients and Healers in the Context of Culture: An Exploration of the Borderland Between Anthropology, Medicine, and Psychiatry* (Berkeley: University of California Press, 1980); Arthur Kleinman, Leon Eisenberg, and Byron Good, "Culture, Illness, and Care: Clinical Lessons from Anthropological and Cross-Cultural Research," *Annals of Internal Medicine* 88, no. 3 (1978): 251–258.

58. Despite all this institutionalization, there was still widespread ambiguity and disagreement about the purpose and instructive capacities of cultural competence. Angela Jenks, "From 'List of Traits' to 'Openmindedness': Emerging Issues in Cultural Competence Education," *Culture, Medicine and Psychiatry* 35, no. 2 (2011): 211. Not only was there heterogeneity in content, but there was also a large degree of variability in commitment to cultural competence. According to the self-described cultural competence experts, cultural competence measures must consistently negotiate the tension between relevance, on the one hand, and theoretical accuracy, on the other. Joseph R. Betancourt and Alexander R. Green, "Commentary: Linking Cultural Competence Training to Improved Health Outcomes: Perspectives From the Field." *Academic Medicine* 85, no. 4 (2010): 583–585; Lauren D. Olsen, "'We'd Rather Be Relevant Than Theoretically Accurate': Translational Medicine and the Transmutation of Cultural Anthropology for Clinical Practice," *Social Problems* 68, no. 3 (2021): 761–777. Critics of the institutionalized cultural competence curriculum and protocols "have pointed to an essentialized, static notion of culture that is conflated with racial and ethnic categories, seen to exist only among exotic 'Others,' and ultimately places blame for health disparities on the 'difference' of culturally marked patients." Jenks, "From 'List

of Traits' to 'Openmindedness,'" 211; Brenda Beagan, "Teaching Social and Cultural Awareness to Medical Students: 'It's All Very Nice to Talk About It in Theory, but Ultimately It Makes No Difference," *Academic Medicine* 78, no. 6 (2003): 605–614; Joseph Gregg and Somnath Saha, "Losing Culture on the Way to Competence: The Use and Misuse of Culture in Medical Education," *Academic Medicine* 81, no. 6 (2006): 542–547; Renee Fox, "Becoming a Physician: Cultural Competence and the Culture of Medicine," *New England Journal of Medicine* 353, no. 13 (2005): 1316–1319; Laurence Kirmayer, "Cultural Competence and Evidence-Based Practice in Mental Health: Epistemic Communities and the Politics of Pluralism," *Social Science and Medicine* 75, no. 3 (2012): 249–256; Janelle Taylor, "Confronting 'Culture' in Medicine's 'Culture of No Culture,'" *Academic Medicine* 7, no. 6 (2003): 555–559; Delese Wear, "Insurgent Multiculturalism: Rethinking How and Why We Teach Culture in Medical Education," *Academic Medicine* 78, no. 6 (2003): 549–554; Joseph Betancourt, Cultural Competence and Medical Education: Many Names, Many Perspectives, One Goal," *Academic Medicine* 81, no. 4 (2002): 499–501.

59. McKinlay and Marceau, "The End of the Golden Age;" Howard Becker, Blanche Geer, Everett C. Hughes, and Anselm C. Strauss, *Boys in White: Student Culture in Medical School* (Chicago: University of Chicago Press, 1961); Robert K. Merton, George G. Reader, and Patricia L. Kendall, *The Student-Physician: Introductory Studies in the Sociology of Medical Education* (Cambridge, MA: Harvard University Press, 1957).

60. Tania M. Jenkins et al., "The Resurgence of Medical Education in Sociology: A Return to Our Roots and an Agenda for the Future," *Journal of Health and Social Behavior* 62, no. 3 (2021): 255–270.

61. Freidson, *Profession of Medicine*; Abbott, *The Systems of the Professions*.

62. Maria Athina Martimianakis, Barret Michalec, Justin Lam, Carrie Cartmill, Janelle S. Taylor, and Frederic W. Hafferty, "Humanism, the Hidden Curriculum, and Educational Reform: A Scoping Review and Thematic Analysis," *Academic Medicine* 90, no. 11 (2015): S5–S13.

63. David J. Flinders, Nel Noddings, and Stephen J. Thornton, "The Null Curriculum: Its Theoretical Basis and Practical Implications, *Curriculum Inquiry* 16, no. 1 (1986): 33–42.

64. Donald W. Light, "Toward a New Sociology of Medical Education," *Journal of Health and Social Behavior* 29, no. 3 (1988): 307–322; Alexandra H. Vinson, "'Constrained Collaboration': Patient Empowerment Discourse as Resource for Countervailing Power," *Sociology of Health and Illness* 38, no. 8 (2016): 1364–1378.

65. "Social practices are ways of doing and thinking that are often tacit, acquire meaning from widely shared presuppositions and underlying semiotic codes, and are tied to particular locations in the social structure and to the collective history of groups. Collective enactment of such practices produces and reproduces those structures and groups." Neil Gross, "A Pragmatist Theory of Social Mechanisms," *American Sociological Review* 74, no. 3 (2009): 359. See also Olga Amsterdamska, "Practices, People, and Places," in *The Handbook of Science and Technology Studies*, ed. Edward J. Hackett, Olga Amsterdamska, Michael Lynch, and Judy Wajcman (Cambridge, MA: MIT Press, 2008), 205–210; Charles Camic, Michele Lamont, and Neil Gross, *Social Knowledge in the Making* (Chicago: University of Chicago Press, 2011).

66. Katherine K. Chen, *Enabling Creative Chaos: The Organization Behind the Burning Man Event* (Chicago: University of Chicago Press, 2009); Thomas Medvetz, *Think Tanks in America* (Chicago: University of Chicago Press, 2012).

67. Legal scholar Leah Goodridge theorizes how professionalism is a racial construct deployed to maintain the white supremacist status quo in the legal profession. She states: "Professionalism as a racial construct manifests itself in two ways. First, that professionalism is measured by how well a person adapts to a hostile work environment is in [and] of itself a racial construct because that system is built for people of color to fail. Second, that professionalism incorporates the ideology to have a thick skin manifests as a racial construct because even the definition of thick skin aligns with who holds the most power . . . The expectation to exhaust all remedies before filing a complaint under the rule effectively operates to force individuals to withstand bias and discrimination for a longer period of time than they would if they immediately sought relief. The abusive conduct is deprioritized, and the burden is placed on the complainant to prove that they tolerated a sufficient amount of it." Leah Goodridge, "Professionalism as a Racial Construct," *UCLA Law Review Discussion (Law Meets World)* 69 (2022): 42,46.

   As Goodridge describes, professionalism serves white interests in how it is conceptualized (e.g., what is professional?) and when it is invoked (e.g., who is professional?)—not only is not wearing one's hair in a particular way seen as unprofessional but also standing up for oneself in the face of brazen racism is seen that way, too. "Professional projects" is Magali Larson's term to capture the contingent nature of professionalization. Trotter has argued that the medical profession's ability to secure its legitimacy and market power was "grounded in embodying a hegemonic, elite white masculinity." Lacking what Trotter refers to as "curative authority," the leaders of the medical profession in the United States then looked for other sources of authority to boost their status—specifically the cultural authority of elite, white men. LaTonya J. Trotter, "A Dream Deferred: Professional Projects as Racial Projects in US Medicine," in *The Routledge Handbook on the American Dream*, ed. Robert C. Hauhart and Mitja Sardoc (New York: Routledge, 2022), 331–351.

68. The history of the medical profession is a history of it being consolidated and reified as a "white institutional space." Glenn E. Bracey and Wendy Leo Moore, "'Race Tests': Racial Boundary Maintenance in White Evangelical Churches," *Sociological Inquiry* 87, no. 2 (2017).

69. Bleakley, "Introduction: The Medical Humanities;" Anne Whitehead and Angela Woods, *The Edinburgh Companion to the Critical Medical Humanities* (Edinburgh: Edinburgh University Press, 2016).

2. PROFESSION-WIDE CURRICULAR DREAMS

1. Tracy Moniz et al., "The Prism Model: Advancing a Theory of Practice for Arts and Humanities in Medical Education," *Perspectives on Medical Education* 10, no. 4 (2021): 207–214; Magda Osman, Bella Eacott, and Suzy Willson, "Arts-Based Interventions in Healthcare Education," *Medical Humanities* 44, no. 1 (2018): 28–33.

2. Before gaining admission into medical school, medical students must fulfill a large number of requirements to be competitive applicants, such as undergraduate courses, high GPA, high MCAT scores, clinical experience, research experience, and volunteer work. Katherine Y. Lin et al., "What Must I Do to Succeed? Narratives from the US Premedical Experience," *Social Science and Medicine* 119 (2014): 98–105. See also Matthew K. Grace, "Subjective Social Status and Premedical Students' Attitudes Towards Medical School," *Social Science and Medicine* 184 (2017): 84–98; Barret Michalec et al., "It's Happening Sooner Than You Think: Spotlighting the Premedical Realm(s)," *Medical Education* 52, no. 4 (2018): 359–361.

3. Tania M. Jenkins, *Doctors' Orders: The Making of Status Hierarchies in an Elite Profession* (New York: Columbia University Press, 2020).

4. American Association of Medical Colleges (AAMC), "Total Enrollment by U.S. Medical School and Race/Ethnicity, 2017–2018," vol. 3, *FACTS: Applicants, Matriculants, Enrollment, Graduates, MD-PhD, and Residency Applicants Data* (Washington, DC: AAMC, 2018).

5. Tania M. Jenkins, Grace Franklyn, Joshua Klugman, and Shalini T. Reddy, "Separate but Equal? The Sorting of USMDs and Non-USMDs in Internal

Medicine Residency Programs," *Journal of General Internal Medicine* 35 (2020): 1458–1464.

6. Institute of Medicine, Committee on Quality of Health Care in America, *Crossing the Quality Chasm: A New Health System for the 21st Century* (Washington, DC: National Academy Press, 2001).

7. Thomas A. LaVeist et al., "The Economic Burden of Racial, Ethnic, and Educational Health Inequities in the US," *Journal of the American Medical Association* 329, no. 19 (2023): 1682–1692.

8. Titilayo Afolabi et al., "Student-Led Efforts to Advance Anti-Racist Medical Education," *Academic Medicine* 96, no. 6 (2021): 802–807, doi:10.1097/ACM .0000000000004043, PMID: 33711839; White Coats 4 Black Lives, "Racial Justice Report Card," accessed May 4, 2018, http://whitecoats4blacklives.org /wp-content/uploads/2018/04/WC4BL-Racial-Justice-Report-Card-2018 -Full-Report-2.pdf.

9. Alexandra H. Vinson and Kelly Underman, "Clinical Empathy as Emotional Labor in Medical Work," *Social Science and Medicine* 251 (2020): 1–9.

10. Liselotte N. Dyrbye et al., "Burnout Among U.S. Medical Students, Residents, and Early Career Physicians Relative to the General U.S. Population," *Academic Medicine* 89, no. 3 (2014): 443–451; Tait D. Shanafelt et al., "Changes in Burnout and Satisfaction with Work-Life Balance in Physicians and the General U.S. Working Population Between 2011 and 2014," *Mayo Clinic Proceedings* 90, no. 12 (2015): 1600–1613; Colin P. West, Tait D. Shanafelt, and Joseph C. Kolars, "Quality of Life, Burnout, Educational Debt, and Medical Knowledge Among Internal Medicine Residents," *Journal of the American Medical Association* 306, no. 9 (2011): 952–960.

11. According to Tracey Collett et al., the Todd report "required that students be introduced, firstly to the rules of sociological observation and analysis; second, to the nature of sociological theories about the rules governing group behavior; and third, to empirical research to test such theories." Tracey Collett, Lauren Brooks, and Simon Forrest, "The History of Sociology Teaching in United Kingdom (UK) Undergraduate Medical Education: An Introduction and Rallying Call," *MedEdPublish* 5 (2016): 152. The Todd report's impact was significant because thirty-two of thirty-four UK medical schools were teaching sociology after its publication, as opposed to just two before.

12. Darrell G. Kirch, "A Word from the President: MCAT 2015: An Open Letter to Pre-Med Students," *AAMC Reporter* (March 2021). In 2008, the AAMC convened the MR5 Committee to conduct the fifth review and revision of the MCAT. The last edition of the exam was launched in 1991, and the updated

examination appeared in 2015 with four main sections. The first two test the applicants' knowledge and use of concepts in biology, chemistry, physics, biochemistry, cellular and molecular biology, research methods, and statistics. The second two test the applicants' knowledge, use, and critical analysis of behavioral and sociocultural determinants of health, sociology, psychology, ethics, philosophy, cross-cultural studies, and population health.

13. Andrew Abbott, *The Systems of the Professions: An Essay on the Division of Expert Labor* (Chicago: University of Chicago Press, 1988); Eliot Freidson, *Profession of Medicine: A Study of the Sociology of Applied Knowledge* (New York: Dodd, Mead, 1970).

14. Alice O'Connor, *Poverty Knowledge: Social Science, Social Policy, and the Poor in Twentieth-Century U.S. History* (Princeton, NJ: Princeton University Press, 2001); Louise Seamster and Victor Ray, "Against Teleology in the Study of Race: Toward the Abolition of the Progress Paradigm," *Sociological Theory* 36, no. 4 (2018): 315–342.

15. Helen H. Small, *The Value of the Humanities* (New York: Oxford University Press, 2016).

16. Rick Rylance, *Literature and the Public Good* (New York: Oxford University Press, 2010), 6.

17. Jeremy Greene, MD-PhD, Johns Hopkins, from an August 15, 2017, AAMC press release by Sarah Mann entitled "Focusing on Arts, Humanities to Develop Well-Rounded Physicians."

18. Most educators I spoke to—clinical, humanist, or social scientist—wished there were more content from the social sciences and humanities; however, Dr. Li was more of an exception to his cohort of educators with his residency placement within a department of social medicine. Most clinical faculty members who were in charge of instruction did not have a dedicated department for the study and application of social sciences or humanities in medicine.

19. William C. McGaghie, "Assessing Readiness for Medical Education: Evolution of the Medical College Admission Test," *Journal of the American Medical Association* 288, no. 9 (2002): 1085–1090.

20. Sociologist Courtney Boen has noted the perils of these approaches: "the downstream consequences of structural racism . . . can promote a form of methodological individualism that focuses on individuals and groups experiencing racism, discrimination, exploitation, and violence, rather than on the institutional actors and systemic processes upholding racism and doing the oppressing, discriminating, and exploiting." Courtney Boen, "Opening

Remarks," *Methods Matter: Understanding and Measuring Race and Racism in Health Research*, Leonard Davis Institute, University of Pennsylvania, September 19, 2023.

21. David J. Doukas, Lawrence B. McCullough, and Stephen E. Wear, "Reforming Medical Education in Ethics and Humanities by Finding Common Ground with Abraham Flexner," *Academic Medicine* 85, no. 2 (2010): 318–323.

22. This finding that the humanities were not seen as core curriculum was consistent with a broad review of how humanism has been conceptualized in the *Academic Medicine* literature over the last thirty years, where even though the humanities and humanism are often conflated, rarely do educators conceptualize the humanities as fundamental to the core learning objectives of medical students (Martiamiakis, Maria A. et al. 2015).

23. Elizabeth Bromley and Joel Braslow, "Teaching Critical Thinking in Psychiatric Training: A Role for the Social Sciences," *American Journal of Psychiatry* 165, no. 11 (2008): 1396–1401; Rita Charon, "Narrative Medicine: A Model for Empathy, Reflection, Profession, and Trust," *Journal of the American Medical Association* 286, no. 15 (2001): 1897–1902; Jonathan M. Metzl and Helena Hansen, "Structural Competency: Theorizing a New Medical Engagement with Stigma and Inequality," *Social Science and Medicine* 103, no. 1 (2014): 126–133.

24. Katarina Wegar, "Sociology in American Medical Education Since the 1960s: The Rhetoric of Reform," *Social Science and Medicine* 35, no. 8 (1992): 959–965.

25. According to *U.S. News and World Report*, around nine allopathic medical schools have a fifth or more of their admissions coming from humanities or social sciences majors. These allopathic medical schools, from lowest (19 percent) to highest (38 percent), are: University of Colorado, George Washington University, Thomas Jefferson University, University of Maryland, University of Pennsylvania, University of Vermont, University of New Mexico, Mount Sinai, Brown University. An additional tenth school is an osteopathic medical school, Michigan State University College of Osteopathic Medicine. Ilana Kowarksi, "10 Medical Schools for Nonscience Majors," *U.S. News & World Report*, 2022, https://www.usnews.com/education/best-graduate-schools/top-medical-schools/slideshows/medical-schools-where-humanities-and-social-sciences-majors-often-attend?onepage.

26. Derrick A. Bell Jr., "Brown v. Board of Education and the Interest-Convergence Dilemma," *Harvard Law Review* 93, no. 3 (1980): 518–533; Elle Lett et al., "Health Equity Tourism: Ravaging the Justice Landscape," *Journal of Medical Systems* 46, no. 17 (2022): 1–21

27. Laura E. Hirshfield, Rachel Yudkowsky, and Yoon Soo Park, "Pre-Medical Majors in the Humanities and Social Sciences: Impact on Communication Skills and Specialty Choice," *Medical Education* 53, no. 4 (2019): 408–416; Lauren D. Olsen and Hana Gebremariam, "Disciplining Empathy: Differences in Empathy with U.S. Medical Students by College Major," *Health: An Interdisciplinary Journal for the Social Study of Health, Illness and Medicine* 26, no. 4 (2022): 475–494; Scott D. Stonington et al., "Case Studies in Social Medicine: Attending to Structural Forces in Clinical Practice," *New England Journal of Medicine* 379, no. 19 (2018): 1958–1961.

3. DESIGNING CURRICULAR PRACTICES AT EACH MEDICAL SCHOOL

1. Frank Dobbin and Alexandra Kalev, "Architecture of Inclusion: Evidence from Corporate Diversity Programs," *Harvard Journal of Law and Gender* 30, no. 2 (2007): 279–301.
2. Organizational sociologist Lauren Edelman coined the term "symbolic compliance" to capture when "ambiguous principles that give organizations the latitude to construct the meaning of compliance in a way that responds to both environmental demands and managerial interests." When an organization, in this case, a medical school, enacts symbolic compliance, they are taking actions that could be interpreted as fulfilling the mandate of the new law or standard, but these actions are limited in power, scope, and effect. Lauren B. Edelman, "Legal Ambiguity and Symbolic Structures: Organizational Mediation of Civil Rights Law," *American Journal of Sociology* 97, no. 6 (1992): 1531.
3. Bridges 2011 Moya Bailey, "The Flexner Report: Standardizing Medical Students Through Region-, Gender-, and Race-Based Hierarchies," *American Journal of Law and Medicine* 43 (2017): 209–223; Rana Hogarth, *Medicalizing Blackness: Making Racial Difference in the Atlantic World, 1780–1840* (Raleigh: University of North Carolina Press, 2017); Deidre Cooper Owens, *Medical Bondage: Race, Gender, and the Origins of American Gynecology* (Athens: University of Georgia Press, 2017); LaTonya J. Trotter, "A Dream Deferred: Professional Projects as Racial Projects in US Medicine," in *The Routledge Handbook on the American Dream* (New York: Routledge, 2022), 331–351; Christopher Willoughby, *Masters of Health: Racial Sciences and Slavery in U.S. Medical Schools* (Raleigh: University of North Carolina Press, 2022).

4. Tania M. Jenkins, "Dual Autonomies, Divergent Approaches: How Stratification in Medical Education Shapes Approaches to Patient Care," *Journal of Health and Social Behavior* 59, no. 2 (2018): 268–282

5. Andrew Abbott, *The Systems of the Professions: An Essay on the Division of Expert Labor* (Chicago: University of Chicago Press, 1988); Eliot Freidson, *Profession of Medicine: A Study of the Sociology of Applied Knowledge* (New York: Dodd, Mead, 1970); Paul Starr, *The Social Transformation of American Medicine* (New York: Basic Books, 1982).

6. Michael D. Cohen, James G. March, and Johan P. Olsen, "A Garbage Can Model of Organizational Choice," *Administrative Science Quarterly* 17, no. 1 (1972): 1–25; Thomas Medvetz, *Think Tanks in America* (Chicago: University of Chicago Press, 2012); Josh Seim, *Bandage, Sort, and Hustle: Ambulance Crews on the Front Lines of Urban Suffering* (Berkeley: University of California Press, 2020).

7. Guian McKee, *Hospital City, Healthcare Nation: Race, Capital, and the Costs of American Healthcare* (Philadelphia: University of Pennsylvania Press, 2023).

8. According to Charlie Eaton and Mitchell L. Stevens, the university is "an organization charged with producing, certifying, and housing knowledge as embodied in artifacts, practices and human beings (faculty), and transferring that knowledge across generations through teaching and research training for adults." Charlie Eaton and Mitchell L. Stevens, "Universities as Peculiar Organizations," *Sociology Compass* 14, no. 3 (2020): 2. Medical schools are places that are fragmented and polysemic, where students learn, where doctors produce knowledge, and where patients are treated.

9. Association of American Medical Colleges (AAMC), "Faculty Roster, December 31, 2021 Snapshot" (Washington, DC: AAMC, 2021).

10. Of the 191,512 full-time faculty across U.S. allopathic medical schools in 2021, there were 19,730 basic scientists; 170,116 clinical faculty; and 1,666 other faculty, 147 of which are social scientists. AAMC, "Faculty Roster, December 31, 2021 Snapshot."

11. Elle Lett, Whitney U. Orji, and Ronnie Sebro, "Declining Racial and Ethnic Representation in Clinical Academic Medicine: A Longitudinal Study of 16 US Medical Specialties," *PLOS One* 13, no. 11 (2018): 1–21.

12. Christopher L. Bennett, Raquel Y. Salinas, Joseph J. Locasio, and Edward W. Boyer, "Two Decades of Little Change: An Analysis of U.S. Medical School Basic Science Faculty by Sex, Race/Ethnicity, and Academic Rank," *PLOS One* 15, no. 7 (2020): e0235190.

13. When operating under time pressures, biases are more likely to happen. Irena Stepanikova, "Racial-Ethnic Biases, Time Pressure, and Medical Decisions,"

Journal of Health and Social Behavior 53, no. 3 [2010]: 329–343. When engaging in hiring or admissions-related decision making, leaders are more likely to engage in "cultural matching," which means they end up choosing applicants who are more likely to be white, elite, and male. Lauren A. Rivera, *Pedigree: How Elite Students Get Elite Jobs* (Princeton, NJ: Princeton University Press, 2015).

14. Paul J. DiMaggio and Walter Powell, "The Iron Cage Revisited: Institutional Isomorphism and Collective Rationality in Organizational Fields," *American Sociological Review* 48, no. 2 (1983): 147–160.

15. Helen Church and Megan Elizabeth Lincoln Brown, "Rise of the Med-Edists: Achieving a Critical Mass of Non-Practicing Clinicians Within Medical Education," *Medical Education* 56, no. 12 (2022): 1160–1163.

16. Association of American Medical Colleges, "Total Enrollment by U.S. Medical School and Race/Ethnicity, 2017–2018," vol. 3, *FACTS: Applicants, Matriculants, Enrollment, Graduates, MD-PhD, and Residency Applicants Data* (Washington, DC: AAMC, 2018). See also Michelle Ko, Mark C. Henderson, and Tonya L. Fancher, "U.S. Medical School Admissions Leaders' Experiences with Barriers to and Advancements in Diversity, Equity, and Inclusion," *Journal of the American Medical Association Network Open* 6, no. 2 (2023): e2254928; Mytien Nguyen, Mayur M. Desai, and Tonya L. Fancher, "Temporal Trends in Childhood Household Income Among Applicants and Matriculants to Medical School and the Likelihood of Acceptance by Income, 2014–2019," *Journal of the American Medical Association* (2023), doi:10.1001/jama.2023.5654; David E. Velasquez, Arman A. Shahriar, and Fidencio Saldana, "Economic Disparity and the Physician Pipeline—Medicine's Uphill Battle." *Journal of General Internal Medicine* (2023), doi:10.1007/s11606-023-08109-3.

17. The mere existence of interprofessional education denotes that it is a problem. See also Ayelet Kuper and Cynthia Whitehead, "The Paradox of Interprofessional Education: IPE as a Mechanism of Maintaining Physician Power?," *Journal of Interprofessional Care* 26, no. 5 (2012): 347–349.

18. Prior work by anthropologists Seth Holmes and Janelle Taylor have critically interrogated the case method and standardized patient as learning devices, calling out their tendencies to depict nonwhite, non-cisgender folks as pathological. See also Christina Amutah et al., "Misrepresenting Race—The Role of Medical Schools in Propagating Physician Bias," *New England Journal of Medicine* 384 (2021): 872–878; Angela Jenks, "From 'List of Traits' to 'Openmindedness': Emerging Issues in Cultural Competence Education," *Culture, Medicine and Psychiatry* 35, no. 2 (2011): 211; Brenda Beagan, "Teaching Social and Cultural Awareness to Medical Students: 'It's All Very Nice to Talk About It in Theory, but Ultimately It Makes No Difference,'" *Academic*

Medicine 78, no. 6 (2003): 605–614; Seth M. Holmes and Maya Pointe, "En-case-ing the Patient: Disciplining Uncertainty in Medical Student Patient Presentations," *Culture Medicine and Psychiatry* 35, no. 1 (2013): 163–182; Janelle Taylor, "Confronting 'Culture' in Medicine's 'Culture of No Culture,'" *Academic Medicine* 7, no. 6 (2003): 555–559.

19. Starting around 2015, there has been an increase in medical journal articles that utilize the "socially complex" phrasing to describe patients from socially marginalized backgrounds, whereas before 2015, the term was used to denote either children navigating the social impacts of autism, communication among health-care workers of different training backgrounds, and interactions among animals that might have more complex social worlds.

20. Natasha K. Warikoo, *The Diversity Bargain: And Other Dilemmas of Race, Admissions, and Meritocracy at Elite Universities* (Chicago: University of Chicago Press, 2016).

21. Paul Hond, "The Hippocratic Overture: Students at Columbia's College of Physicians and Surgeons Are Getting Ready to Practice. Will It Make Them Better Doctors?," *Columbia Magazine* (Spring/Summer 2015): 18–29.

22. Hond, "The Hippocratic Overture."

23. Beyond the more glaring markers of prestige, such as university pedigree, Rivera found that employers were looking for potential hires that could be seen as a "formidable playmate," or someone who would be fun, sociable, well-adjusted—and screening out the boring and bookish nerds. Rivera, *Pedigree*, 95. As Rivera deftly asserts, the signals that the employers look for to identify such candidates (these signals of "authentic passion" and "extraordinary achievement" in "high-status leisure pursuits," like going to the Olympics for fencing, or being a concert cellist) are "associated with white, upper- and upper-middle-class culture." Rivera, *Pedigree*, 99.

24. Michael W. Rabow et al., "Insisting on the Healer's Art: The Implications of Required Participation in a Medical School Course on Values and Humanism," *Teaching and Learning in Medicine* 28, no. 1 (2016): 61–71.

25. Ellen Berrey, *The Enigma of Diversity: The Language of Race and the Limits of Racial Justice* (Chicago: University of Chicago Press, 2015).

4. ENACTING CURRICULAR PRACTICES IN THE CLASSROOM

1. As John Hoberman writes in his history of racism in the medical profession, "this awkwardness about practicing and discussing race relations has long been a fact of medical life the profession has been slow to recognize or deal

with in a deliberate or systematic way." John Hoberman, *Black and Blue: The Origins and Consequences of Medical Racism* (Berkeley: University of California Press, 2012), 2.

2. In a similar example, Dr. Mogin, a white male social scientist, described how he tried to "meet" students "where they are" when teaching them about the social construction perspective by describing how the meanings of illness evolve over time. He went on to say that he was "not some sort of Foucauldian clown and actually fortunate enough to write a book with a neurologist on Alzheimer's and I feel like I can make a pretty strong argument and also know the science which I think is very important when you work in this world." By stating that he was not "Foucauldian clown," Dr. Mogin shows what students were learning but also what was left out.

3. Jonathan M. Metzl and Helena Hansen, "Structural Competency: Theorizing a New Medical Engagement with Stigma and Inequality," *Social Science and Medicine* 103, no. 1 (2014): 126–133.

4. Jonathan Kahn, "Pills for Prejudice: Implicit Bias and Technical Fix for Racism," *American Journal of Law and Medicine* 43 (2017): 263–278.

5. Cultural understandings of race or other social backgrounds have been shown to be dangerous. As lawyer and anthropologist Khiara Bridges notes, "ideas about patients contribute to health disparities . . . cultural stereotypes and beliefs in the way people from certain cultures 'just are' can be just as dangerous—and just as racist—as racism." Khiara M. Bridges, *Reproducing Race: An Ethnography of Pregnancy as a Site of Racialization* (Berkeley: University of California Press, 2011), 131–135. Additional opinion pieces have discussed the silence of medical educators around race as a topic (Malika Sharma and Ayelet Kuper, "The Elephant in the Room: Talking Race in Medical Education," *Advances in Health Sciences Education* 22, no. 3 [2017]: 762) and the lack of qualified faculty members to teach about the social determinants of health (Barry F. Saunders and Lundy Braun, "Reforming the Use of Race in Medical Pedagogy," *American Journal of Bioethics* 17, no. 9 [2017]: 51), thus pointing to clinical faculty members as untrained and uncertain about how to teach social sciences. Some critical race scholars engaged in medical education write that "current medical pedagogy lacks self-reflexivity; encodes social identities like race and gender as essential risk factors; neglects to examine root causes of health inequity; and fails to teach learners how to challenge injustice." Jennifer Tsai, Edwin Lindo, and Khiara Bridges, "Seeing the Window, Finding the Spider: Applying Critical Race Theory to Medical Education to Make Up Where Biomedical Models and Social

Determinants of Health Curricula Fall Short," *Frontiers in Public Health* 9 (2021): 1–10. Hoberman refers to this type of cultural approach to race as physicians' "playing anthropologist," where clinical faculty members engage in an "amateur cultural anthropology that acquaints the physician with the lives of his patients," which is a reiterated version of past medical racism where "a curiosity about the anatomy of the racial alien and a sense of entitlement that confers a right to examine her body for evidence of racial difference." Hoberman, *Black and Blue*, 55–56.

Joe Kai, Ruth Bridgewater, and John Spencer, "'Just Think of TB and Asians,' That's All I Ever Hear': Medical Learners' Views About Training to Work in an Ethnically Diverse Society," *Medical Education* 35, no. 3 (2001): 250–256; Kelsey Ripp and Lundy Braun, "Race/Ethnicity in Medical Education: An Analysis of a Question Bank for Step 1 of the USMLE," *Teaching and Learning in Medicine* 29, no. 2 (2017): 115–122; Saunders and Braun, "Reforming the Use of Race in Medical Pedagogy;" Sharma and Kuper, "The Elephant in the Room;" Jennifer Tsai, Neil Baldwin, Laura Ucik, Christopher Hasslinger, and George Paul, "Race Matters? Examining and Rethinking Race Portrayal in Preclinical Medical Education," *Academic Medicine* 91, no. 7 (2016): 916–920; Jennifer Tsai, Edwin Lindo, and Khiara Bridges, "Seeing the Window, Finding the Spider: Applying Critical Race Theory to Medical Education to Make Up Where Biomedical Models and Social Determinants of Health Curricula Fall Short," *Frontiers in Public Health* 9 (2021): 1–10.

6. Christina Amutah et al., "Misrepresenting Race—The Role of Medical Schools in Propagating Physician Bias," *New England Journal of Medicine* 384, no. 9 (2021): 872–878; Saunders and Braun, "Reforming the Use of Race in Medical Pedagogy;" Warwick Anderson, "Teaching Race at Medical School: Social Scientists on the Margin," *Social Studies of Science* 38, no. 5 (2008): 785–800.

7. Ruha Benjamin, "Cultura Obscura: Race, Power, and 'Culture Talk' in the Health Sciences." *American Journal of Law and Medicine* 43 (2017): 225–238. "Culture talk" was initially posed by Mahmood Mamdani in "Good Muslim, Bad Muslim: A Political Perspective on Culture and Terrorism," *American Anthropologist* 104, no.3 (2002): 766–775, as "the predilection to define cultures according to their presumed 'essential' characteristics."

8. Faith E. Fletcher, Folasade C. Lapite, and Alicia Best, "Rethinking the Moral Authority of Experience: Critical Insights and Reflections from Black Women Scholars," *The American Journal of Bioethics* 23, no. 1 (2023): 27–30.

9. Brooke A. Cunningham et al., "Physicians' Anxiety Due to Uncertainty and Use of Race in Medical Decision Making," *Medical Care* 52, no. 8 (2014): 728–733; Michelle van Ryn et al., "The Impact of Racism on Clinician Cognition, Behavior, and Clinical Decision Making," *DuBois Review* 8, no. 1 (2011): 199–218.

10. Jamie L. Manzer and Ann V. Bell, "We're a Little Biased: Medicine and the Management of Bias Through the Case of Contraception," *Journal of Health and Social Behavior* 62, no. 2 (2021): 120–135.

11. Rita Charon and Martha Montello, *Stories Matter: The Role of Narrative in Medical Ethics* (New York: Routledge, 2004); Rita Charon, "What to Do with Stories: The Sciences of Narrative Medicine," *Canadian Family Physician* 53, no. 8 (2007): 1265–1267.

12. Eva Illouz, *Saving the Modern Soul: Therapy, Emotions, and the Culture of Self-Help* (Berkeley: University of California Press, 2008).

13. Alexandra H. Vinson and Kelly Underman, "Clinical Empathy as Emotional Labor in Medical Work," *Social Science and Medicine* 251 (2020): 1–9; Allison J. Pugh, "Emotions and the Systematization of Connective Labor," *Theory, Culture & Society* 39, no. 5 (2021): 23–42.

14. Sara Carmel and Seymour M. Glick, "Compassionate-Empathic Physicians: Personality Traits and the Social-Organizational Factors That Enhance or Inhibit This Behavior Pattern," *Social Science and Medicine* 43, no. 8 (1996): 1253–1261; Eric B. Larson and Xin Yao, "Clinical Empathy as Emotional Labor in the Patient-Physician Relationship," *Journal of the American Medical Association* 293, no. 9 (2005): 1100; Reidar Pedersen, "Empathy Development in Medical Education: A Critical Review," *Medical Teaching* 32, no. 7 (2010): 593–600; Kelly Underman, *Feeling Medicine: How the Pelvic Exam Shapes Medical Training* (New York: New York University Press, 2020); Vinson and Underman, "Clinical Empathy as Emotional Labor."

15. Alexandra H. Vinson, "'Constrained Collaboration': Patient Empowerment Discourse as Resource for Countervailing Power," *Sociology of Health and Illness* 38, no. 8 (2016): 1364–1378.

16. Underman, *Feeling Medicine*, 18; Vinson and Underman, "Clinical Empathy as Emotional," 3

17. See the latest "synergistic" partnership between the Gold Foundation and Medallia, one of their corporate sponsors, in creating a commodified tool to "measure" humanistic care. Stacy Bodziak, "Gold and Medallia Build a New Tool to Measure Humanistic Care," *Gold Foundation News*, May 19, 2023.

18. Nguemeni Tiako, Max Jordan, Eugenia C. South, and Victor Ray, "Medical Schools as Racialized Organizations: A Primer," *Annals of Internal Medicine* 174, no. 8 (2022): 1143–1144.

19. With an entire section of the website dedicated to "profiles in creativity," this group is an exercise in showcasing the immense talents of artistic physicians. This description appears in the visual arts section: "Delicate Touch in Painting Translates to Ophthamology. Artist Statement: Dr. Jaclyn Gurwin, a third year Opthamology resident at the University of Pennsylvania's Scheie Eye Institute, has been drawing and painting since a young age. As a fine arts minor at the University of Pennsylvania, she received a formal art training that helped hone visual and technical skills that have since been very helpful in her medical career." It is precisely this "fine art" training from a young age that is touted by medical school leadership. Jaclyn Gurwin, "Delicate Touch in Painting Translates to Ophthalmalogy," Doctors Who Create, January 19, 2019, https://www.doctorswhocreate.com/delicate-touch-in-painting-translates-to-ophthalmology.

20. These books include: *Healing: When A Nurse Becomes a Patient* by Theresa Brown (WW, RN); *The Beauty of Dusk: On Vision Lost and Found* by Frank Bruni (WM, NYT columnist); *The Deep Places: A Memoir of Illness and Discovery* by Ross Douthat (WM, NYT columnist); *Every Deep-Drawn Breath: A Critical Care Doctor on Healing Recovery, and Transforming Medicine in the ICU* by Wesley Ely (WM, MD); *Left on Tenth: A Second Chance at Life* by Delia Ephron (WW, writer); *The Urge: History of Addiction* by Carl Erik Fisher (WM, MD); *The Facemaker: A Visionary Surgeon's Battle to Mend the Disfigured Soldiers of WWI* by Lindsey Fitzharris (WW, writer with PhD); *The Invisible Kingdom: Reimagining Chronic Illness* by Meghan O'Rourke (WW, writer/editor of Yale Law Review); *Write for Your Life* by Anna Quindlen (WW, writer); *Just Human: The Quest for Disability Wisdom, Respect, and Inclusion* by Arielle Silverman (WW, PhD); *Under the Skin: The Hidden Toll of Racism on American Lives and on the Health of Our Nation* by Linda Villarosa (BW, journalist); *The Song of Our Scars: The Untold Story of Pain* by Haider Warraich (MoC, MD).

5. RECEIVING CURRICULAR PRACTICES

1. Thomas F. O'Connell et al., "A National Longitudinal Survey of Medical Students' Intentions to Practice Among the Underserved," *Academic Medicine* 93, no. 1 (2018): 90–97; Sean M. Phelan et al., "The Effects of Racism

in Medical Education on Students' Decisions to Practice in Underserved or Minority Communities," *Academic Medicine* 94, no. 8 (2019): 1178–1189.

2. Other scholars have captured the heteronormativity in medical education. Marie Murphy, "Hiding in Plain Sight: The Production of Heteronormativity in Medical Education," *Journal of Contemporary Ethnography* 45, no. 3 (2014): 256–289; Juno Obedin-Maliver et al., "Lesbian, Gay, Bisexual, and Transgender–Related Content in Undergraduate Medical Education," *Journal of the American Medical Association* 306, no. 9 (2011): 971–977.

3. Another example of how clinical relevance was on everyone's minds comes from Dr. Sampson, a white female humanist, who recounted this humorous misunderstanding that occurred the first time she proposed doing a small elective on literature. She said, "When I started to tell my colleagues, I think I'm going to do something with literature, there was this rush of enthusiasm. Everybody was so excited, I was like 'whoa really this is great.' They said, '[Y]eah we really need someone who can explain EBM to our students—like, evidence-based medicine.' So they thought I was talking about literature reviews."

4. Alexandra Vinson, in her ethnographic research, has shown medical students equate belonging within the profession with the possession of biomedical knowledge and technical expertise. Alexandra H. Vinson, "Teaching the Work of Doctoring: How the Medical Profession Adapts to Change" (PhD diss., University of California San Diego, 2015); Alexandra H. Vinson, "'Constrained Collaboration': Patient Empowerment Discourse as Resource for Countervailing Power," *Sociology of Health and Illness* 38, no. 8 (2016): 1364–1378; Alexandra H. Vinson, "Short White Coats: Knowledge, Identity, and Status Negotiations of First-Year Medical Students," *Symbolic Interaction* 42, no. 3 (2019): 395–411.

5. Tiffany D. Joseph and Laura E. Hirshfield, "'Why Don't You Get Somebody New to Do It?' Race and Cultural Taxation in the Academy," *Ethnic and Racial Studies* 34, no. 1 (2011): 121–141; Veronica Lerma, Laura T. Hamilton, Kelly Nielsen, "Racialized Equity Labor, University Appropriation, and Student Resistance," *Social Problems* 67, no. 2 (2020): 286–303; Barret Michalec, Tina Martimianakis, Jon Tilburt, and Frederic W. Hafferty, "Why It's Unjust to Expect Location-Specific, Language-Specific, or Population-Specific Service from Students with Underrepresented Minority or Low-Income Backgrounds," *AMA Journal of Ethics* 19, no. 3 (2017): 238–244; Amado M. Padilla, "Ethnic Minority Scholars, Research, and Mentoring: Current and Future Issues," *Educational Researcher* 23, no. 4 (1994): 24–27.

6. Angelique M. Davis and Rose Ernst, "Racial Gaslighting," *Politics, Groups, and Identities* 7, no. 4 (2019): 763.

7. Physicians tend to be unwilling to be whistleblowers and are disciplined to handle things "in-house." John Hoberman, *Black and Blue: The Origins and Consequences of Medical Racism* (Berkeley: University of California Press, 2012), 9. See also Charles L. Bosk, *Forgive and Remember: Managing Medical Failure* (Chicago: University of Chicago Press, 1979); Katherine C. Kellogg, *Challenging Operations: Medical Reform and Resistance in Surgery* (Chicago: University of Chicago Press, 2011).

8. Mary Blair-Loy and Erin Cech, *Misconceiving Merit: Paradoxes of Excellence and Devotion in Academic Science and Engineering* (Chicago: University of Chicago Press, 2022).

9. Basil Bernstein, "Class, Codes and Control: Towards a Theory of Educational Transmissions," *British Journal of Educational Studies* 25, no. 1 (1977): 28. See also Kelly Underman's new work on burnout: Kelly Underman, "Burnout Inventories and the Unsettled Science of Wellness in Health Professions Education," BeSST Conference, Edinburgh, August 27, 2023.

10. Foucault's concept of "technologies of the self" is instructive here because it captures the ways in which we work on ourselves—this work might be physical, moral, emotional—and oriented toward transforming ourselves to attain particular objectives, like "happiness, purity, wisdom, perfection or immortality." Technologies of self are a form of power and, as an extension of it, governmentality is a set of practices or techniques that are organized and oriented around governing subjects. "Art of government" is an achievement of medical educators because it is the biopolitical control of their students by getting them to govern themselves. Michel Foucault, *Technologies of the Self: A Seminar with Michel Foucault*, ed. Luther H. Martin, Huck Gutman, and Patrick Hutton (Amherst: University of Massachusetts Press, 1988), 18.

11. Knowledge is cultural material—written standards, disease diagrams, novels, artwork, music, disparities data—that serves as "hermeneutic devices helping us make sense of the world but also as cultural devices that tap into, elicit, and channel complex emotional apparatuses (such as indignation, compassion, longing for love, fear, and anxiety)." Eva Illouz, *Saving the Modern Soul: Therapy, Emotions, and the Culture of Self-Help* (Berkeley: University of California Press, 2008), 18.

12. Shamus Rahman Khan, *Privilege: The Making of an Adolescent Elite at St. Paul's School* (Princeton, NJ: Princeton University Press, 2011).

13. Frederic W. Hafferty, "Cadaver Stories and the Emotional Socialization of Medical Students," *Journal of Health and Social Behavior* 29, no. 4 (1988): 344–356; Vinson, "Short White Coats."

14. Shamus R. Khan, *Privilege: The Making of an Adolescent Elite at St. Paul's School* (Princeton, NJ: Princeton University Press, 2011).

15. Elites hold "vastly disproportionate control" over scarce, valued resources that can be used to gain access to material or symbolic advantages in society." Khan, *Privilege*, 290. In medical education, this can occur through what Jenkins calls status separation—where the prestige of MD rises to the top over other medical degrees. Tania M. Jenkins, *Doctors' Orders: The Making of Status Hierarchies in an Elite Profession* (New York: Columbia University Press, 2020).

CONCLUSION

1. Charles Goodwin, "Professional Vision," in *Aufmerksamkeit: Geschichte-Theorie-Empirie* (Wiesbaden: Springer Fachmedien Wiesbaden, 2015), 387–425.

2. Elan Burton et al., "Assessment of Bias in Patient Safety Reporting Systems Categorized by Physician Gender, Race and Ethnicity, and Faculty Rank," *Journal of the American Medical Association Network Open* 5, no. 5 (2022): e2213234; Brooke A. Cunningham et al., "Physicians' Anxiety Due to Uncertainty and Use of Race in Medical Decision Making," *Medical Care* 52, no. 8 (2014): 728–733.

3. Frank Dobbin and Alexandra Kalev, "Architecture of Inclusion: Evidence from Corporate Diversity Programs," *Harvard Journal of Law and Gender* 30, no. 2 (2007): 279–301.

4. Maralynn Bann, Savannah Larimore, Jessica Wheeler, and Lauren D. Olsen, "Implementing a Social Determinants of Health Curriculum in Undergraduate Medical Education: A Qualitative Analysis of Faculty Experience," *Academic Medicine* 97, no. 11 (2022): 1665–1672; Malika Sharma, Andrew D. Pinto, Arno K. Kumagai, "Teaching the Social Determinants of Health: A Path to Equity or a Road to Nowhere?," *Academic Medicine* 93, no. 1 (2018): 25–30.

5. Jamie L. Manzer and Ann V. Bell, "We're a Little Biased: Medicine and the Management of Bias Through the Case of Contraception," *Journal of Health and Social Behavior* 62, no. 2 (2021): 120–135. See also Eeva Sointu, "'Good' Patient/'Bad' Patient: Clinical Learning and the Entrenching of Inequality," *Sociology of Health and Illness* 39, no. 1 (2017): 63–77.

6. Many members of the medical profession engage in "race aversive" practices, characterized by silence and evasion. John Hoberman, *Black and Blue: The Origins and Consequences of Medical Racism* (Berkeley: University of California Press, 2012), 208.

7. Shamus R. Khan, *Privilege: The Making of an Adolescent Elite at St. Paul's School* (Princeton, NJ: Princeton University Press, 2011).

8. The conceptualization of the humanities as providing therapeutic benefits in the Western tradition dates to Aristotle, who thought that the humanities allowed individuals to explore the human condition; poetry's therapeutic benefits were extolled by John Stuart Mill when he happened upon some poetry during an existential crisis as a young utilitarian. From Sir Philip Sidney, writing about 1580, in *The Defense of Poesy*, painting the intrinsic value of the humanities as that which "preserves and transmits the past and its achievements, both intellectual and artistic to the present . . . teaches and delights . . . strengthens virtue and morals" (Sir Philip Sidney, "The Defense of Poesy," in *The Defense of Poesy Otherwise Known as an Apology for Poetry*, ed. Albert S. Cook (Boston: Ginn, 1890), cited in Rick Rylance, *Literature and the Public Good* [New York: Oxford University Press, 2010], 60), to former U.S. President Barack Obama, quoted in the *New York Times* Review of Books in 2015 as saying that literature teaches one "to be comfortable that the world is complicated . . . that it is possible to connect with someone else even though they are different from you," the intrinsic value of the humanities extends beyond the therapeutic benefits detailed in this dissertation chapter on the therapeutic curriculum.

9. Goodley Dan and Rebecca Lawthom, "Critical Disability Studies, Brexit and Trump: A Time of Neoliberal-Ableism," *Rethinking History* 23, no. 2 (2019): 235.

10. Scott Frickel, Sahra Gibbon, Jeff Howard, Joanna Kempner, Gwen Ottinger, and David J. Hess, "Undone Science: Charting Social Movement and Civil Society Challenges to Research Agenda Setting," *Science, Technology, and Human Values* 35, no. 4 (2010): 464.

11. Scott Frickel and Kelly Moore, *The New Political Sociology of Science: Institutions, Networks, and Power* (Madison: University of Wisconsin Press, 2006), 56.

12. A parallel example will be helpful to illustrate this point. In their study of a translational neuro lab, Caragh Brosnan and Mike Michael point to the necessity of the clinician-scientist as the critical bridge, or "knowledge broker" to these "cultural" divides. Caragh Brosnan and Mike Michael, "Enacting the 'Neuro' in Practice: Translational Research, Adhesion and the Promise of Porosity," *Social Studies of Science* 44, no. 5 (2014): 680–700. See also Justin Waring et al., *An Ethnographic Study of Knowledge Sharing Across the Boundaries Between Care Processes, Services, and Organizations: The Contributions to 'Safe' Hospital Discharge*. Health Services and Delivery Research No. 2.29 (London: National Institute for Health Research, 2014). Acting as a pivotal facilitator of translational work, this "hybrid professional" provides a platform for understanding the active work that individual academic actors must engage in to realize the objectives of their translational projects. Mike Michael, Steven Wainwright,

and Clare Williams, "Temporality and Prudence: On Stem Cells as 'Phronesic Things'," *Configurations* 13, no. 3 (2005): 386.

13. Deborah Gordon contends that physicians find the merits of clinical experience outweigh biomedical knowledge, which are borne out in the actual practice of clinical medicine. She argues that, within medicine, "intuition, based on vast concrete experience, is the hallmark of expertise" in clinical settings Deborah Gordon, "Clinical Science and Clinical Expertise: Changing Boundaries Between Art and Science in Medicine," in *Biomedicine Examined*, ed. Margaret Lock and Deborah Gordon (Amsterdam: Kluwer-Academic, 1988), 258. In a study of physicians' work environments that complicates Gordon's finding, Daniel Menchik and David Meltzer found that the prestige of physicians' work environments—in this case, hospitals—affected how esteem was allocated to physicians. Daniel Menchik and David Meltzer, "The Cultivation of Esteem and Retrieval of Scientific Knowledge in Physician Networks," *Journal of Health and Social Behavior* 51, no. 1 (2010): 137–152. Hospitals, for Menchik and Meltzer, "each contain their own social structures of reputation and expertise that influence how medicine is practiced, regardless of the guidelines and scientific research in a field." Menchik and Meltzer, "The Cultivation of Esteem," 138. At low-prestige hospitals, physicians could be held in high esteem by their colleagues if they were well read in clinical medicine; however, at high-prestige hospitals, the pedigree of the physician held more weight in designations of high esteem.

14. Katherine C. Kellogg, *Challenging Operations: Medical Reform and Resistance in Surgery* (Chicago: University of Chicago Press, 2011); Charles L. Bosk, *Forgive and Remember: Managing Medical Failure* (Chicago: University of Chicago Press, 1979).

15. LaTonya J. Trotter has argued that the medical profession's ability to secure its legitimacy and market power was "grounded in embodying a hegemonic, elite white masculinity." Lacking what Trotter refers to as "curative authority," the leaders of the medical profession in the United States then looked for other sources of authority to boost their status—specifically the cultural authority of elite, white men. LaTonya J. Trotter, "A Dream Deferred: Professional Projects as Racial Projects in US Medicine," in *The Routledge Handbook on the American Dream*, ed. Robert C. Hauhart and Mitja Sardoc (New York: Routledge, 2022), 333.

16. Anthony Ryan Hatch, "The Data Will Not Save Us: Afropessimism and Racial Antimatter in the COVID-19 Pandemic," *Big Data and Society* 9, no. 1 (2022): 1–13.

17. California Department of Justice, *Report and Recommendations* (Sacramento, CA: Office of the Attorney General, 2019), 53.

18. Ellen Berrey, *The Enigma of Diversity: The Language of Race and the Limits of Racial Justice* (Chicago: University of Chicago Press, 2015).

19. Rita Charon, "Narrative Medicine: A Model for Empathy, Reflection, Profession, and Trust," *Journal of the American Medical Association* 286, no. 15 (2001): 1897–1902; Rita Charon, "What to Do with Stories: The Sciences of Narrative Medicine," *Canadian Family Physician* 53, no. 8 (2007): 1265–1267; Rita Charon and Martha Montello, *Stories Matter: The Role of Narrative in Medical Ethics* (New York: Routledge, 2004).

20. When educators install critical curricular practices into their medical school, it is an accomplishment, as "new knowledge fields are fundamentally political outcomes, the result of struggles for resources, identities, and status." Jerry A. Jacobs and Scott Frickel, "Interdisciplinarity: A Critical Assessment," *Annual Review of Sociology* 35 (2009): 57.

21. Frickel and Moore, *The New Political Sociology of Science.*

22. Jennifer C. Mueller, "Racial Ideology or Racial Ignorance? An Alternative Theory of Racial Cognition," *Sociological Theory* 38, no. 2 (2020): 145–146; Charles W. Mills, *The Racial Contract* (Ithaca, NY: Cornell University Press, 1997).

23. Medical school leaders in the United Kingdom, for example, are tackling a more critical approach to learning about social inequalities head on, with their decolonizing the curriculum movement. One article published by educators from the University of College London (UCL), for example pointed to three central lines of change, going "from a colonial to decolonial lens." The first is in the domain of epistemology, where they move from the dominance of biomedical ways of knowing toward a more "epistemic pluralism," where they in turn engage in critiques of positivism and uplift non-Western healing modalities and interdisciplinary perspectives. The second is oriented around how medical educators approach teaching diversity in which they move from what they term "cultural destructiveness"—that is, the stereotyping or disparaging of non-Western, nonwhite cultures—toward one of "cultural safety," which requires medical educators and students alike to practice critical reflection and cultural humility. The third domain is in the scope of the curriculum, where the UCL educators move from "sanctioned ignorance," which is an apt term to describe the curricular designers' decisions to exclude topics on structural inequality, toward a critical consciousness that takes the historical and contemporary examination of the medical profession and societies seriously. They summarize their approach with

some overarching themes, which are markedly different from the way most U.S. clinical faculty members approach medical education that they are worth mentioning. Thematically, the UCL educators wish to confront the hierarchies, Eurocentrism, and stratification in their institution and profession while embracing a focus on equity, decentering, and intersectionality. Sarah H. M. Wong, Faye Gishen, Amali U. Lokugamage, "'Decolonizing the Medical Curriculum': Humanizing Medicine Through Epistemic Pluralism, Cultural Safety, and Critical Consciousness," *London Review of Education* 19, no. 1 (2021), doi:10.14324/LRE.19.1.16.

METHODOLOGICAL APPENDIX: DATA SOURCES AND RESEARCH DESIGN

1. Oscar E. Dimant, Tiffany E. Cook, Richard E. Green, and Asa E. Radix, "Experiences of Transgender and Gender Nonbinary Medical Students and Physicians," *Transgender Health* 4, no. 1 (2019): 209–216; Josef Madrigal, Sarah Rudasil, Zachary Tran, Jonathan Bergman, and Peyman Benharash, "Sexual and Gender Minority Identity in Undergraduate Medical Education: Impact on Experience and Career Trajectory," *PLoS One* 16, no. 11 (2021): e0260387; Jules L. Madzia, "Inequality in Medical Professionalization and Specialization" (PhD diss., University of Cincinnati, 2023).

2. Stacy J. Williams, Laura Pecenco, and Mary Blair-Loy, "Medical Professions: The Status of Women and Men," (La Jolla, CA: University of California San Diego, 2013)

3. Association of American Medical Colleges (AAMC), "Diversity in Medical Education: Facts and Figures 2016," Vol. 6, *Facts and Figures Report* (Washington, DC: AAMC, 2016).

4. Janet K. Shim, *Heart-Sick: The Politics of Risk, Inequality, and Heart Disease* (New York: New York University Press, 2014).

5. Shim, *Heart-Sick*.

6. Ann Morning, *The Nature of Race: How Scientists Think and Teach About Human Difference* (Berkeley: University of California Press, 2011).

7. Shim, *Heart-Sick*.

8. Aviad Raz and Judith Fadlon, "'We Came to Talk with the People Behind the Disease': Communication and Control in Medical Education," *Culture, Medicine and Psychiatry* 30, no. 1 (2006): 55–75.

9. Michael Omi and Howard Winant, *Racial Formation in the United States: From the 1960s to the 1990s* (New York: Routledge, 1994).

10. Morning, *The Nature of Race*.

11. Kathy Charmaz, *Constructing Grounded Theory: A Practical Guide Through Qualitative Analysis* (Thousand Oaks, CA: Sage, 2006).

12. Titilayo Afolabi et al., "Student-Led Efforts to Advance Anti-Racist Medical Education," *Academic Medicine* 96, no. 6 (2021): 802–807, doi:10.1097/ACM.0000000000004043, PMID: 33711839; Christina Amutah et al., "Misrepresenting Race—The Role of Medical Schools in Propagating Physician Bias," *New England Journal of Medicine* 384, no. 9 (2021): 872–878; Jennifer Tsai, Neil Baldwin, Laura Ucik, Christopher Hasslinger, and George Paul, "Race Matters? Examining and Rethinking Race Portrayal in Preclinical Medical Education," *Academic Medicine* 91, no. 7 (2016): 916–920; White Coats 4 Black Lives, "Racial Justice Report Card," accessed May 4, 2018, http://whitecoats4blacklives.org/wp-content/uploads/2018/04/WC4BL-Racial-Justice-Report-Card-2018-Full-Report-2.pdf.

13. Tania M. Jenkins, *Doctors' Orders: The Making of Status Hierarchies in an Elite Profession* (New York: Columbia University Press, 2020).

14. Brooke A. Cunningham et al., "Physicians' Anxiety Due to Uncertainty and Use of Race in Medical Decision Making," *Medical Care* 52, no. 8 (2014): 728–733; Ning Hsieh and stef. m. shuster, "Health and Health Care of Sexual and Gender Minorities," *Journal of Health and Social Behavior* 62, no. 2 (2021): 318–333; Sean M. Phelan et al., "The Effects of Racism in Medical Education on Students' Decisions to Practice in Underserved or Minority Communities," *Academic Medicine* 94, no. 8 (2019): 1178–1189; stef m. shuster, *Trans Medicine: The Emergence and Practice of Treating Gender* (New York: New York University Press, 2021).

BIBLIOGRAPHY

Abbott, Andrew. *The Systems of the Professions: An Essay on the Division of Expert Labor*. Chicago: University of Chicago Press, 1988.

Afolabi, Titilayo, Hannah M. Borowsky, Daniella M. Cordero, Dereck W. Paul Jr., Jordan T. Said, Raquel S. Sandoval, Denise Davis, Daniele Ölveczky, and Avik Chatterjee. "Student-Led Efforts to Advance Anti-Racist Medical Education." *Academic Medicine* 96, no. 6 (2021): 802–807, doi:10.1097/ACM.0000000000004043, PMID: 33711839.

Ahmed, Sara. *Complaint!* Durham, NC: Duke University Press, 2021.

Albert, Mathieu, Elise Paradis, and Ayelet Kuper. "Interdisciplinary Promises Versus Practices in Medicine: The Decoupled Experiences of Social Sciences and Humanities Scholars." *Social Science and Medicine* 126, no. 1 (2015): 17–25.

Amsterdamska, Olga. "Practices, People, and Places." In *The Handbook of Science and Technology Studies*, ed. Edward J. Hackett, Olga Amsterdamska, Michael Lynch, and Judy Wajcman, 205–210. Cambridge, MA: MIT Press, 2008.

Amutah, Christina, Kaliya Greenidge, Adjoa Mante, Michelle Munyikwa, Sanjna Surya, Eve Higginbotham, David S. Jones, Risa Lavizzo-Mourey, Dorothy Roberts, Jennifer Tsai, and Jaya Aysola. "Misrepresenting Race—The Role of Medical Schools in Propagating Physician Bias." *New England Journal of Medicine* 384 (2021): 872–878.

Anderson, Warwick. "Teaching Race at Medical School: Social Scientists on the Margin." *Social Studies of Science* 38, no. 5 (2008): 785–800.

Antelby, Michel. *Manufacturing Morals: The Values of Silence in Business School Education*. Chicago: University of Chicago Press, 2013.

Arragon, Rex F. "Humanities and Medical Education." *Journal of Medical Education* 35, no. 10 (1960): 908–912.

Arum, Richard, and Josipa Roksa. *Academically Adrift: Limited Learning on College Campuses.* Chicago: University of Chicago Press, 2011.

Association of American Medical Colleges. *Cultural Competence Education for Medical Students.* Washington, DC: AAMC, 2005.

Association of American Medical Colleges. "Diversity in Medical Education: Facts and Figures 2016." Vol. 6, *Facts and Figures Report.* Washington, DC: AAMC, 2016.

Association of American Medical Colleges. *Faculty Roster, December 31, 2021 Snapshot.* Washington, DC: AAMC, 2021.

Association of American Medical Colleges. "Matriculating Student Questionnaire." Washington, DC: AAMC, 2016.

Association of American Medical Colleges. "Report of the Joint Committee on the Teaching of the Social and Environmental Factors in Medicine." *Minutes of the Proceedings of the Fifty-Seventh Annual Meeting Held in Edgewater Park, Mississippi.* Chicago: AAMC, 1946.

Association of American Medical Colleges. "Total Enrollment by U.S. Medical School and Race/Ethnicity, 2017–2018." Vol. 3, *FACTS: Applicants, Matriculants, Enrollment, Graduates, MD-PhD, and Residency Applicants Data.* Washington, DC: AAMC, 2018.

Association of American Medical Colleges. *U.S. Medical School Deans by Dean Type and Race/Ethnicity.* Washington DC: AAMC, 2023.

Bagdley, Robin F., and Samuel W. Bloom. "Behavioral Sciences and Medical Education: The Case of Sociology." *Social Science and Medicine* 7, no. 1 (1973): 923–941.

Bailey, Moya. "The Flexner Report: Standardizing Medical Students Through Region-, Gender-, and Race-Based Hierarchies." *American Journal of Law and Medicine* 43 (2017): 209–223.

Balmer, Andrew S., Jane Calvert, Claire Marris, Susan Molyneux-Hodgson, Emma Frow, Matthew Kearnes, Kate Bulpin, Pablo Schyfter, Adrian Mackenzie, and Paul Martin. "Taking Roles in Interdisciplinary Collaborations: Reflections on Working in Post-ELSI Spaces in the UK Synthetic Biology Community." *Science and Technology Studies* 28, no. 3 (2015): 3–25.

Bann, Maralynn, Savannah Larimore, Jessica Wheeler, and Lauren D. Olsen. "Implementing a Social Determinants of Health Curriculum in Undergraduate Medical Education: A Qualitative Analysis of Faculty Experience." *Academic Medicine* 97, no. 11 (2022): 1665–1672.

Beagan, Brenda. "Teaching Social and Cultural Awareness to Medical Students: 'It's All Very Nice to Talk About It in Theory, but Ultimately It Makes No Difference.'" *Academic Medicine* 78, no. 6 (2003): 605–614.

Becker, Howard, Blanche Geer, Everett C. Hughes, and Anselm C. Strauss. *Boys in White: Student Culture in Medical School*. Chicago: University of Chicago Press, 1961.

Bell, Derrick A., Jr. "Brown v. Board of Education and the Interest-Convergence Dilemma." *Harvard Law Review* 93, no. 3 (1980): 518–533.

Benjamin, Ruha. "Catching Our Breath: Critical Race STS and the Carceral Imagination." *Engaging Science, Technology, and Society* 2, no. 1 (2016): 145–156.

Benjamin, Ruha. "Cultura Obscura: Race, Power, and 'Culture Talk' in the Health Sciences." *American Journal of Law and Medicine* 43 (2017): 225–238.

Bennett, Christopher L., Raquel Y. Salinas, Joseph J. Locasio, and Edward W. Boyer. "Two Decades of Little Change: An Analysis of U.S. Medical School Basic Science Faculty by Sex, Race/Ethnicity, and Academic Rank." *PLOS One* 15, no. 7 (2020): e0235190.

Benneworth, Paul, and Ben W. Jongbloed. "Who Matters to Universities? A Stakeholder Perspective on Humanities, Arts, and Social Sciences Valorization." *Higher Education* 59, no. 5 (2010): 567–588.

Berman, Elizabeth Popp. "Explaining the Move Toward the Market in US Academic Science: How Institutional Logics Can Change Without Institutional Entrepreneurs." *Theory and Society* 41, no. 3 (2012): 261–299.

Berman, Elizabeth Popp. "Not Just Neoliberalism: Economization in US Science and Technology." *Science, Technology and Human Values* 39, no. 3 (2014): 397–431.

Bernstein, Basil. "Class, Codes and Control: Towards a Theory of Educational Transmissions." *British Journal of Educational Studies* 25, no. 1 (1977): 1–28.

Berrey, Ellen. *The Enigma of Diversity: The Language of Race and the Limits of Racial Justice*. Chicago: University of Chicago Press, 2015.

Berry, Sarah, Therese Jones, and Erin Lamb. "Editors' Introduction: Health Humanities: The Future of Pre-Health Education Is Here." *Journal of Medical Humanities* 38 (2017): 353–360.

Betancourt, Joseph R. and Alexander R. Green. "Commentary: Linking Cultural Competence Training to Improved Health Outcomes: Perspectives From the Field." *Academic Medicine* 85, no. 4 (2010): 583–585.

Betancourt, Joseph. "Cultural Competence and Medical Education: Many Names, Many Perspectives, One Goal." *Academic Medicine* 81, no. 4 (2002): 499–501.

Binder, Amy J. *Contentious Curricula: Afrocentrism and Creationism in American Public Schools*. Princeton, NJ: Princeton University Press, 2002.

Binder, Amy J. "Why Do Some Curricular Challenges 'Work' While Others Do Not? The Case of Three Afrocentric Challenges: Atlanta, Washington DC, and New York State." *Sociology of Education* 73, no. 1 (2000): 69–91.

Blair-Loy, Mary. *Competing Devotions: Career and Family Among Women Executives.* Cambridge, MA: Harvard University Press, 2005.

Blair-Loy, Mary, and Erin Cech. *Misconceiving Merit: Paradoxes of Excellence and Devotion in Academic Science and Engineering.* Chicago: University of Chicago Press, 2022.

Bleakley, Alan. "Introduction: The Medical Humanities: A Mixed Weather Front on a Global Scale." In *Routledge Handbook of the Medical Humanities*, ed. Alan Bleakley. New York: Routledge, 2019.

Bloom, Samuel W. "The Role of the Sociologist in Medical Education." *Journal of Medical Education* 34, no. 7 (1959): 667–673.

Bloom, Samuel W. "Structure and Ideology in Medical Education: An Analysis of Resistance to Change." *Journal of Health and Social Behavior* 29, no. 2 (1988): 294–306.

Bloom, Samuel W. *The Word as Scalpel: History of Medical Sociology.* Oxford: Oxford University Press, 2002.

Bodziak, Stacy. "Gold and Medallia Build a New Tool to Measure Humanistic Care." *Gold Foundation News*, May 19, 2023.

Boelen, Charles, and Jeffrey E. Heck. *Defining and Measuring the Social Accountability of Medical Schools.* Geneva: World Health Organization, 1995.

Boen, Courtney. "Opening Remarks." *Methods Matter: Understanding and Measuring Race and Racism in Health Research.* Leonard Davis Institute, University of Pennsylvania, September 29, 2023.

Borrego, Maura, and Lynita K. Newswander. "Definitions of Interdisciplinary Research: Toward Graduate-Level Interdisciplinary Learning Outcomes." *The Review of Higher Education* 34, no. 1 (2010): 61–84.

Bosk, Charles L. *Forgive and Remember: Managing Medical Failure.* Chicago: University of Chicago Press, 1979.

Bosk, Charles L. *The Price of Perfection.* Baltimore, MD: Eastern Sociological Society, 2023.

Bostick, Nathan, Karine Morin, Regina Benjamin, and Daniel Higginson. "Physicians' Ethical Responsibilities in Addressing Racial and Ethnic Healthcare Disparities." *Journal of the National Medical Association* 98, no. 8 (2006): 1329–1334.

Bracey, Glenn E., and Wendy Leo Moore. "'Race Tests': Racial Boundary Maintenance in White Evangelical Churches." *Sociological Inquiry* 87, no. 2 (2017): 282–302.

Bridges, Khiara M. *Reproducing Race: An Ethnography of Pregnancy as a Site of Racialization.* Berkeley: University of California Press, 2011.

Brint, Steven. *The Future of the City of Intellect: The Changing American University.* Palo Alto, CA: Stanford University Press, 2002.

Brint, Steven, Mark Riddle, Lori Turk-Bicakci, and Charles S. Levy. "From the Liberal to the Practical Arts in American Colleges and Universities: Organizational Analysis and Curricular Change." *The Journal of Higher Education* 76, no. 2 (2005): 151–180.

Brintnall, Michael. *National Endowment for the Humanities, Public Witness Testimony Submitted to the Interior, Environment, and Related Agencies Subcommittee.* Committee on Appropriations, U.S. House of Representatives, House Congressional Testimony, 2012. www.nhalliance.org/advocacy/testimony/congressional-testimony-fy-2012-neh.shtml.

Brody, Howard. "Defining the Medical Humanities: Three Conceptions and Three Narratives." *Journal of Medical Humanities* 32 (2011): 1–7.

Bromley, Elizabeth, and Joel Braslow. "Teaching Critical Thinking in Psychiatric Training: A Role for the Social Sciences." *American Journal of Psychiatry* 165, no. 11 (2008): 1396–1401.

Brooks, Peter. *The Humanities and Public Life.* New York: Fordham University Press, 2015.

Brosnan, Caragh, and Mike Michael. "Enacting the 'Neuro' in Practice: Translational Research, Adhesion and the Promise of Porosity." *Social Studies of Science* 44, no. 5 (2014): 680–700.

Brown, Phil, Brian Mayer, Stephen Zavestoski, Theo Luebke, Joshua Mandelbaum, and Sabrina McCormick. "The Health Politics of Asthma: Environmental Justice and Collective Illness Experience in the United States." *Social Science and Medicine* 57, no. 3 (2003): 453–464.

Brown, Theresa. *Healing: When A Nurse Becomes a Patient.* Chapel Hill: Algonquin Books, 2022.

Brown, Tony N. "Being Black and Feeling Blue: The Mental Health Consequences of Racial Discrimination." *Race and Society* 2, no. 2 (2000): 117–131.

Bruni, Frank. *The Beauty of Dusk: On Vision Lost and Found.* New York: Simon and Schuster, 2023.

Brunsma, David L., David G. Embrick, and Jean H. Shin. "Graduate Students of Color: Race, Racism, and Mentoring in the White Waters of Academia." *Sociology of Race and Ethnicity* 3, no. 1 (2017): 1–13.

Burns, Chester. "History in Medical Education: The Development of Current Trends in the United States." *Bulletin of the New York Academy of Medicine* 51, no. 7 (1975): 851–869.

Burton, Elan, Brenda Flores, Barbara Jerome, Yan Min, Yvonne A. Maldonado, and Malai Fassioto. "Assessment of Bias in Patient Safety Reporting Systems Categorized by Physician Gender, Race and Ethnicity, and Faculty Rank." *Journal of the American Medical Association Network Open* 5, no. 5 (2022): e2213234.

Byrd, W. Michael, and Linda A. Clayton. "Race, Medicine and Healthcare in the United States: A Historical Survey." *Journal of the National Medical Association* 93, no. 3 (2001): 11–34.

Byrd, W. Michael, and Linda A. Clayton. *An American Health Dilemma*, vol. 2. *Race, Medicine, and Healthcare in the U.S. 1900–2000*. New York: Routledge, 2002.

Cadbury, William E., Jr., Charles Dawson, Thomas Hunter, and Richard Masland. "The Responsibility of the Arts College to the Student Planning the Study of Medicine." *Journal of the Association of American Medical Colleges* 26, no. 3 (1951): 169–171.

California Department of Justice. *Report and Recommendations*. Sacramento, CA: Office of the Attorney General, 2019.

Camic, Charles, Michele Lamont, and Neil Gross. *Social Knowledge in the Making*. Chicago: University of Chicago Press, 2011.

Carmel, Sara, and Seymour M. Glick. "Compassionate-Empathic Physicians: Personality Traits and the Social-Organizational Factors That Enhance or Inhibit This Behavior Pattern." *Social Science and Medicine* 43, no. 8 (1996): 1253–1261.

Casalino, Lawrence P. "Unfamiliar Tasks, Contested Jurisdictions: The Changing Organization Field of Medical Practice in the United States." *Journal of Health and Social Behavior* 45, Special Issue (2004): S59–S75.

Casberg, Melvin A. "Medical Education Takes Inventory." *Journal of the Association of American Medical Colleges* 25, no. 5 (1950): 306–311.

Charmaz, Kathy. *Constructing Grounded Theory: A Practical Guide Through Qualitative Analysis*. Thousand Oaks, CA: Sage, 2006.

Charon, Rita. "Narrative Medicine: A Model for Empathy, Reflection, Profession, and Trust." *Journal of the American Medical Association* 286, no. 15 (2001): 1897–1902.

Charon, Rita. "What to Do with Stories: The Sciences of Narrative Medicine." *Canadian Family Physician* 53, no. 8 (2007): 1265–1267.

Charon, Rita, and Martha Montello. *Stories Matter: The Role of Narrative in Medical Ethics*. New York: Routledge, 2004.

Chen, Katherine K. *Enabling Creative Chaos: The Organization Behind the Burning Man Event*. Chicago: University of Chicago Press, 2009.

Church, Helen, and Megan Elizabeth Lincoln Brown. "Rise of the Med-Ed-Ists: Achieving a Critical Mass of Non-Practicing Clinicians Within Medical Education." *Medical Education* 56, no. 12 (2022): 1160–1163.

Clark, Burton R. *The Higher Education System: Academic Organization in Cross-National Perspective*. Berkeley: University of California Press, 1983.

Clarke, Adele E., Janet K. Shim, Laura Mamo, Jennifer Ruth Fosket, and Jennifer R. Fishman. "Biomedicalization: Technoscientific Transformations of Health,

Illness, and U.S. Biomedicine." *American Sociological Review* 68, no. 2 (2003): 161–194.

Cohen, Michael D., James G. March, and Johan P. Olsen. "A Garbage Can Model of Organizational Choice." *Administrative Science Quarterly* 17, no. 1 (1972): 1–25.

Collett, Tracey, Lauren Brooks, and Simon Forrest. "The History of Sociology Teaching in United Kingdom (UK) Undergraduate Medical Education: An Introduction and Rallying Call." *MedEdPublish* 5 (2016): 152.

Collins, Harry, and Robert Evans. *Rethinking Expertise.* Chicago: University of Chicago Press, 2007.

Committee on Educating Health Professionals to Address the Social Determinants of Health; Board on Global Health, Institute of Medicine, National Academies of Sciences, Engineering, and Medicine. *A Framework for Educating the Health Professionals to Address the Social Determinants of Health.* Washington, DC: National Academies Press, 2016.

Conant, James B. "College Education for the Future Doctor." Speech delivered February 13, 1939, Folder 277, Dean's Subject File, Harvard Medical Archives, Rare Books Department, Countway Library, Harvard Medical School, Boston, 1939.

Cottom, Tressie McMillan. *Thick: And Other Essays.* New York: The New Press, 2018.

Coulehan, Jack. "What Is Medical Humanities and Why?" *Literature Arts and Medicine Magazine,* January 25, 2008, https://medhum.med.nyu.edu/magazine/archives/100.

Cunningham, Brooke A., Vence L. Bonham, Sherril L. Sellers, Hsin-Chieh Yeh, and Lisa Cooper. "Physicians' Anxiety Due to Uncertainty and Use of Race in Medical Decision Making." *Medical Care* 52, no. 8 (2014): 728–733.

Cyrus, Kali D. "Medical Education and the Minority Tax." *Journal of the American Medical Association* 317, no. 18 (2017): 1833–1834.

Davis, Angelique M., and Rose Ernst. "Racial Gaslighting." *Politics, Groups, and Identities* 7, no. 4 (2019): 761–774.

DelVecchio Good, Mary Jo, Cara James, Byron J. Good, and Anne E. Becker. "The Culture of Medicine and Racial, Ethnic and Class Disparities in Health." Working Paper 199, Russell Sage Foundation, 2002.

Diez-Roux, Ana V., and Christina Mair. "Neighborhoods and Health." *Annals of the New York Academy of the Sciences* 1186, no. 1 (2010): 125–145.

DiMaggio, Paul J., and Walter Powell. "The Iron Cage Revisited: Institutional Isomorphism and Collective Rationality in Organizational Fields." *American Sociological Review* 48, no. 2 (1983): 147–160.

Dimant, Oscar E., Tiffany E. Cook, Richard E. Green, and Asa E. Radix. "Experiences of Transgender and Gender Nonbinary Medical Students and Physicians." *Transgender Health* 4, no. 1 (2019): 209–216.

Dobbin, Frank, and Alexandra Kalev. "Architecture of Inclusion: Evidence from Corporate Diversity Programs." *The Harvard Journal of Law and Gender* 30, no. 2 (2007): 279–301.

Dolan, Brian. "History, Medical Humanities, and Medical Education." *Social History of Medicine* 23, no. 2 (2010): 393–405.

Donoghue, Frank. *The Last Professors: The Corporate University and the Fate of the Humanities*. Bronx, NY: Fordham University Press, 2008.

Doukas, David J., Lawrence B. McCullough, and Stephen E. Wear. "Reforming Medical Education in Ethics and Humanities by Finding Common Ground with Abraham Flexner." *Academic Medicine* 85, no. 2 (2010): 318–323.

Douthat, Ross. *The Deep Places: A Memoir of Illness and Discovery*. New York: Convergent Books, 2021.

Dyrbye, Liselotte N., Colin P. West, Daniel Satele, Sonja Boone, Litjen Tan, Jeff Sloan, and Tait D. Shanafelt. "Burnout Among U.S. Medical Students, Residents, and Early Career Physicians Relative to the General U.S. Population." *Academic Medicine* 89, no. 3 (2014): 443–451.

Eaton, Charlie, and Mitchell L. Stevens. "Universities as Peculiar Organizations." *Sociology Compass* 14, no. 3 (2020): e12768.

Edelman, Lauren B. "Legal Ambiguity and Symbolic Structures: Organizational Mediation of Civil Rights Law." *American Journal of Sociology* 97, no. 6 (1992): 1531–1576.

Ely, Wesley E. *Every Deep-Drawn Breath: A Critical Care Doctor on Healing, Recovery, and Transforming Medicine in the ICU*. New York, Scribner, 2021.

Engelhardt, H. Tristam. *The Foundations of Bioethics*. Oxford: Oxford University Press, 1986.

Engelhardt, H. Tristram. "Managed Care and the Deprofessionalization of Medicine." *The Ethics of Managed Care: Professional Integrity and Patient Rights*, ed. W. B. Bondeson and J. W. Jones, 93–108. Amsterdam: Kluwer Academic Publishers, 2001.

Ephron, Delia. *Left on Tenth: A Second Chance at Life*. New York: Little, Brown, and Company, 2022.

Epstein, Steven. *Inclusion: The Politics of Difference in Medical Research*. Chicago: University of Chicago Press, 2007.

Evans, John H. *The History and Future of Bioethics: A Sociological View*. Oxford: Oxford University Press, 2012.

Evans, John H. *Playing God? Human Genetic Engineering and the Rationalization of Public Bioethical Debate*. Chicago: University of Chicago Press, 2002.

Evans, John H. "Stratification in Knowledge Production: Author Prestige and the Influence on American Academic Debate." *Poetics* 33, no. 1 (2005): 111–133.

Feagin, Joe R., and Zinobia Bennefield. "Systemic Racism and U.S. Healthcare." *Social Science and Medicine* 103, no. 1 (2014): 7–14.

Fisher, Carl Erik. *The Urge: History of Addiction*. New York Penguin Books, 2022.

Fitzgerald, Des, Melissa M. Littlefield, Kasper J. Knudsen, James Tonks, and Martin J. Dietz. "Ambivalence, Equivocation and the Politics of Experimental Knowledge: A Transdisciplinary Neuroscience Encounter." *Social Studies of Science* 44, no. 5 (2014): 453–473.

Fitzharris, Lindsey. *The Facemaker: A Visionary Surgeon's Battle to Mend the Disfigured Soldiers of WWI*. New York: Farrar, Straus and Giroux, 2022.

Fletcher, Faith E., Folasade C. Lapite, and Alicia Best. "Rethinking the Moral Authority of Experience: Critical Insights and Reflections from Black Women Scholars." *The American Journal of Bioethics* 23, no. 1 (2023): 27–30.

Flexner, Abraham. *Medical Education in the United States and Canada: A Report to the Carnegie Foundation for the Advancement of Teaching*. Bulletin Number Four. New York: Carnegie Foundation, 1910.

Flinders, David J., Nel Noddings, and Stephen J. Thornton. "The Null Curriculum: Its Theoretical Basis and Practical Implications. *Curriculum Inquiry* 16, no. 1 (1986): 33–42.

Foster, Anna, and Kathleen Kendall. "The Experience of Teaching Biomedical Science Subjects to UK Medical Students." [version 1; not peer reviewed]. *MedEdPublish* 13 (2023): 61 (slides), doi:10.21955/mep.1115231.1.

Foucault, Michel. *Technologies of the Self: A Seminar with Michel Foucault*, ed. Luther H. Martin, Huck Gutman, and Patrick Hutton. Amherst: University of Massachusetts Press, 1988.

Fox, Renee. "Becoming a Physician: Cultural Competence and the Culture of Medicine." *New England Journal of Medicine* 353, no. 13 (2005): 1316–1319.

Fox, Renee. "Training for Uncertainty." In *The Student-Physician: Introductory Studies in the Sociology of Medical Education*, ed. Robert K. Merton, George G. Reader, and Patricia L. Kendall, 207–241. Cambridge, MA: Harvard University Press, 1957.

Freidson, Eliot. *Profession of Medicine: A Study of the Sociology of Applied Knowledge*. New York: Dodd, Mead, 1970.

Frickel, Scott, and Kelly Moore. *The New Political Sociology of Science: Institutions, Networks, and Power*. Madison: University of Wisconsin Press, 2006.

Frickel, Scott, Sahra Gibbon, Jeff Howard, Joanna Kempner, Gwen Ottinger, and David J. Hess. "Undone Science: Charting Social Movement and Civil Society Challenges to Research Agenda Setting." *Science, Technology, and Human Values* 35, no. 4 (2010): 444-473.

Gamble, Vanessa N. "Under the Shadow of Tuskegee: African Americans and Healthcare." *American Journal of Public Health* 87, no. 11 (1997): 1773-1778.

Giroux, Henry A., and Anthony N. Penna. "Social Education in the Classroom: The Dynamics of the Hidden Curriculum." *Theory and Research in Social Education* 7, no. 1 (1979): 21-42.

Go, Julian. "Race, Empire, and Epistemic Exclusion: Or the Structures of Sociological Thought." *Sociological Theory* 38, no. 2 (2020): 79-100.

Good, Byron. *Medicine, Rationality, and Experience: An Anthropological Perspective.* Cambridge: Cambridge University Press, 1994.

Goodley, Dan, and Rebecca Lawthom. "Critical Disability Studies, Brexit and Trump: A Time of Neoliberal-Ableism." *Rethinking History* 23, no. 2 (2019): 233-251.

Goodridge, Leah. "Professionalism as a Racial Construct." *UCLA Law Review Discussion (Law Meets World)* 69 (2022): 38-54.

Goodwin, Charles. "Professional Vision." In *Aufmerksamkeit: Geschichte-Theorie-Empirie*, ed. Sabine Reh, Kathrin Berdelmann, and Jorg Dinkelaker, 387-425. Wiesbaden: Springer Fachmedien Wiesbaden, 2015.

Gordon, Deborah. "Clinical Science and Clinical Expertise: Changing Boundaries Between Art and Science in Medicine." In *Biomedicine Examined*, ed. Margaret Lock and Deborah Gordon, 257-295. Amsterdam: Kluwer Academic Publishers, 1988.

Grace, Matthew K. "Subjective Social Status and Premedical Students' Attitudes Towards Medical School." *Social Science and Medicine* 184 (2017): 84-98.

Gravlee, Clarence C. "How Whiteness Works: JAMA and the Refusals of White Supremacy." *Somatosphere*, March 27, 2021. https://somatosphere.com/tag/race/.

Gregg, Joseph, and Somnath Saha. "Losing Culture on the Way to Competence: The Use and Misuse of Culture in Medical Education." *Academic Medicine* 81, no. 6 (2006): 542-547.

Greil, Arthur L., Julia McQuillan, Karina M. Shreffler, Katherine M. Johnson, and Kathleen S. Slauson-Blevins. "Race-Ethnicity and Medical Services for Infertility: Stratified Reproduction in a Population-Based Sample of U.S. Women." *Journal of Health and Social Behavior* 52, no. 4 (2011): 493-509.

Gross, Neil. "A Pragmatist Theory of Social Mechanisms." *American Sociological Review* 74, no. 3 (2009): 358-379.

Gurwin, Jaclyn. "Delicate Touch in Painting Translates to Ophthamalogy." Doctors Who Create, January 19, 2019. https://www.doctorswhocreate.com/category/visual-arts/.

Guttentag, Otto E. "A Course Entitled 'The Medical Attitude': An Orientation in the Foundations of Medical Thought." *Journal of Medical Education* 35, no. 10 (1960): 903–907.

Hackett, Edward J., Olga Amsterdamska, Michael Lynch, and Judy Wajcman, eds. *The Handbook of Science and Technology Studies.* Cambridge, MA: MIT Press, 2008.

Hafferty, Frederic W. "Beyond Curriculum Reform: Confronting Medicine's Hidden Curriculum. *Academic Medicine* 73, no. 1 (1998): 193–197.

Hafferty, Frederic W. "Cadaver Stories and the Emotional Socialization of Medical Students." *Journal of Health and Social Behavior* 29, no. 4 (1988): 344–356.

Hafferty, Frederic W. "Reconfiguring the Sociology of Medical Education: Emerging Topics and Pressing Issues." In *Handbook of Medical Sociology*, 5th ed., ed. Chloe Bird, Peter Conrad, and Allen Fremont, 238–257. Upper Saddle River, NJ: Prentice Hall, 2000.

Hafferty, Frederic W., and Brian Castellani. "The Increasing Complexities of Professionalism." *Academic Medicine* 85, no. 2 (2010): 288–301.

Hafferty, Frederic W., and Ronald Franks. "The Hidden Curriculum, Ethics Teaching, and the Structure of Medical Education." *Academic Medicine* 69, no. 11 (1994): 861–871.

Hafferty, Frederic W., and Joseph F. O'Donnell. *The Hidden Curriculum in Health Professional Education.* Hanover, NH: Dartmouth College Press, 2015.

Hallett, Timothy, and Marc Ventresca. "Inhabited Institutions: Social Interactions and Organizational Forms in Gouldner's *Patterns of Industrial Bureaucracy*." *Theory and Society* 35, no. 2 (2006): 213–236.

Hatch, Anthony Ryan. "The Data Will Not Save Us: Afropessimism and Racial Antimatter in the COVID-19 Pandemic." *Big Data and Society* 9, no. 1 (2022): 1–13.

Haug, Marie R. "A Re-Examination of the Hypothesis of Physician Deprofessionalization." *Milbank Memorial Fund Quarterly* 66, no. 2 (1988): 48–56.

Hirshfield, Laura E., Rachel Yudkowsky, and Yoon Soo Park. "Pre-Medical Majors in the Humanities and Social Sciences: Impact on Communication Skills and Specialty Choice." *Medical Education* 53, no. 4 (2019): 408–416.

Hoberman, John. *Black and Blue: The Origins and Consequences of Medical Racism.* Berkeley: University of California Press, 2012.

Hoffman, Lily M. *The Politics of Knowledge: Activist Movements in Medicine and Planning.* Albany, NY: SUNY Press, 1989.

Hogarth, Rana A. *Medicalizing Blackness: Making Racial Difference in the Atlantic World, 1780–1840.* Raleigh: University of North Carolina Press, 2017.

Holmes, Seth M., Angela Jenks, and Scott Stonington. "Clinical Subjectivation: Anthropologies of Contemporary Biomedical Training." *Culture, Medicine, and Psychiatry* 35, no. 2 (2011): 105–112.

Holmes, Seth M., and Maya Pointe. "En-Case-Ing the Patient: Disciplining Uncertainty in Medical Student Patient Presentations." *Culture Medicine and Psychiatry* 35, no. 1 (2013): 163–182.

Hond, Paul. "The Hippocratic Overture: Students at Columbia's College of Physicians and Surgeons Are Getting Ready to Practice. Will it Make Them Better Doctors?" *Columbia Magazine* Spring/Summer 2015: 18–29.

hooks, bell. *Teaching Community: A Pedagogy of Hope.* New York: Routledge, 2003.

Horton, Mary E. Kollmer. "A (Un)Natural Alliance: Medical Education and the Humanities." PhD diss., Emory University, 2020.

Hsieh, Ning, and stef. m. shuster. "Health and Health Care of Sexual and Gender Minorities." *Journal of Health and Social Behavior* 62, no. 3 (2021): 318–333.

Illouz, Eva. *Saving the Modern Soul: Therapy, Emotions, and the Culture of Self-Help.* Berkeley: University of California Press, 2008.

Institute of Medicine, Committee on Quality of Health Care in America. *Crossing the Quality Chasm: A New Health System for the 21st Century.* Washington, DC: National Academy Press, 2001.

Jackson, Pamela Brayboy, Peggy Thoits, and Howard F. Taylor. "Composition of the Workplace and Psychological Well-Being: The Effects of Tokenism on America's Black Elite." *Social Forces* 74, no. 2 (1995): 543–557.

Jacobs, Jerry A., and Scott Frickel. "Interdisciplinarity: A Critical Assessment." *Annual Review of Sociology* 35 (2009): 43–65.

Jacobsen, Carlyle. "Student Selection Problems: ROUND TABLE A." *Journal of Medical Education* 25, no. 1 (1950): 7–11.

Jenkins, Tania M. *Doctors' Orders: The Making of Status Hierarchies in an Elite Profession.* New York: Columbia University Press, 2020.

Jenkins, Tania M. "Dual Autonomies, Divergent Approaches: How Stratification in Medical Education Shapes Approaches to Patient Care." *Journal of Health and Social Behavior* 59, no. 2 (2018): 268–282.

Jenkins, Tania M., Grace Franklyn, Joshua Klugman, and Shalini T. Reddy. "Separate but Equal? The Sorting of USMDs and Non-USMDs in Internal Medicine Residency Programs." *Journal of General Internal Medicine* 35 (2020): 1458–1464.

Jenkins, Tania M., and Shalini Reddy. "Revisiting the Rationing of Medical Degrees in the United States." *Contexts* 15, no. 4 (2016): 36–41.

Jenkins, Tania M., Kelly Underman, Alexandra H. Vinson, Lauren D. Olsen, and Laura Hirshfield. "The Resurgence of Medical Education in Sociology: A Return to Our Roots and an Agenda for the Future." *Journal of Health and Social Behavior* 62, no. 3 (2021): 255–270.

Jenks, Angela. "From 'List of Traits' to 'Openmindedness': Emerging Issues in Cultural Competence Education." *Culture, Medicine and Psychiatry* 35, no. 2 (2011): 209–235.

Joseph, Tiffany D., and Laura E. Hirshfield. "'Why Don't You Get Somebody New to Do It?' Race and Cultural Taxation in the Academy." *Ethnic and Racial Studies* 34, no. 1 (2011): 121–141.

Kahn, Jonathan. "Pills for Prejudice: Implicit Bias and Technical Fix for Racism." *American Journal of Law and Medicine* 43 (2017): 263–278.

Kai, Joe, Ruth Bridgewater, and John Spencer. "'Just Think of TB and Asians,' That's All I Ever Hear': Medical Learners' Views About Training to Work in an Ethnically Diverse Society." *Medical Education* 35, no. 3 (2001): 250–256.

Karabel, Jerome. *The Chosen: The Hidden History of Admission and Exclusion at Harvard, Yale, and Princeton.* New York: Houghton Mifflin, 2005.

Kellogg, Katherine C. *Challenging Operations: Medical Reform and Resistance in Surgery.* Chicago: University of Chicago Press, 2011.

Khan, Shamus Rahman. *Privilege: The Making of an Adolescent Elite at St. Paul's School.* Princeton, NJ: Princeton University Press, 2011.

Kirch, Darrell G. "A Word from the President: MCAT 2015: An Open Letter to Pre-Med Students." *AAMC Reporter* (March 2012).

Kirmayer, Laurence. "Cultural Competence and Evidence-Based Practice in Mental Health: Epistemic Communities and the Politics of Pluralism." *Social Science and Medicine* 75, no. 3 (2012): 249–256.

Kleinman, Arthur. *Patients and Healers in the Context of Culture: An Exploration of the Borderland Between Anthropology, Medicine, and Psychiatry.* Berkeley: University of California Press, 1980.

Kleinman, Arthur, Leon Eisenberg, and Byron Good. "Culture, Illness, and Care: Clinical Lessons from Anthropological and Cross-Cultural Research." *Annals of Internal Medicine* 88, no. 3 (1978): 251–258.

Ko, Michelle, Mark C. Henderson, and Tonya L. Fancher. "U.S. Medical School Admissions Leaders' Experiences with Barriers to and Advancements in Diversity, Equity, and Inclusion," *Journal of the American Medical Association Network Open* 6, no. 2 (2023): e2254928.

Kowarksi, Ilana. "10 Medical Schools for Nonscience Majors." *U.S. News & World Report.* September 19, 2022. https://www.usnews.com/education/best

-graduate-schools/top-medical-schools/slideshows/medical-schools-where
-humanities-and-social-sciences-majors-often-attend?onepage.

Kuper, Ayelet, and Cynthia Whitehead. "The Paradox of Interprofessional Education: IPE as a Mechanism of Maintaining Physician Power?" *Journal of Interprofessional Care* 26, no. 5 (2012): 347–349.

Larson, Eric B., and Xin Yao. "Clinical Empathy as Emotional Labor in the Patient-Physician Relationship." *Journal of the American Medical Association* 293, no. 9 (2005): 1100–1106.

LaVeist, Thomas A., Eliseo J. Perez-Stable, Patrick Richard, Andrew Anderson, Lydia A. Isaac, Riley Santiago, Celine Okoh, Nancy Breen, Tilda Farhat, Assen Assenov, and Darrell J. Gaskin. "The Economic Burden of Racial, Ethnic, and Educational Health Inequities in the US." *Journal of the American Medical Association* 329, no. 19 (2023): 1682–1692.

Lerma, Veronica, Laura T. Hamilton, and Kelly Nielsen. "Racialized Equity Labor, University Appropriation, and Student Resistance." *Social Problems* 67, no. 2 (2020): 286–303.

Lett, Elle, Dali Adekunle, Patrick McMurray, Emmanuella Ngozi Asabor, Whitney Irie, Melissa A. Simon, Rachel Hardeman, and Monica R. McLemore. "Health Equity Tourism: Ravaging the Justice Landscape." *Journal of Medical Systems* 46, no. 17 (2022): 1–6.

Lett, Elle, Whitney U. Orji, and Ronnie Sebro. "Declining Racial and Ethnic Representation in Clinical Academic Medicine: A Longitudinal Study of 16 US Medical Specialties." *PLOS One* 13, no. 11 (2018): 1–21.

Lewin, Tamar. "As Interest Fades in the Humanities, Colleges Worry." *New York Times*, October 30, 2013.

Liaison Committee on Medical Education. *Functions and Structure of a Medical School: Standards for Accreditation of Medical Education Programs Leading to the MD Degree.* Washington, DC: AAMC, 2018.

Light, Donald W. "Introduction: Ironies of Success—A New History of the American Health Care 'System.'" *Journal of Health and Social Behavior* 45, no. 1 (2004): 1–24.

Light, Donald W. "Introduction: Strengthening Ties Between Specialties and Disciplines." *American Journal of Sociology* 97, no. 4 (1992): 909–918.

Light, Donald W. "The Medical Profession and Organizational Change: From Professional Dominance to Countervailing Power." In *Handbook of Medical Sociology*, ed. Chloe E. Bird, Peter Conrad, and Allen M. Fremont, 210–225. New York: Prentice Hall, 2000.

Light, Donald W. "Toward a New Sociology of Medical Education." *Journal of Health and Social Behavior* 29, no. 3 (1988): 307–322.

Lin, Katherine Y., Renee R. Anspach, Brett Crawford, Sonali Parnami, Andrea Fuhrel-Forbis, and Raymond G. De Vries. "What Must I Do to Succeed? Narratives from the US Premedical Experience." *Social Science and Medicine* 119 (2014): 98–105.

Link, Bruce G., and Jo Phelan. "Social Conditions as Fundamental Causes of Disease." *Journal of Health and Social Behavior*, Extra Issue (1995): 80–94.

Lipsitz, George. "The Possessive Investment in Whiteness: Racialized Social Democracy and the 'White' Problem in American Studies." *American Quarterly* 47, no. 3 (1995): 369–387.

Ludmerer, Kenneth M. *Learning to Heal: The Development of American Medical Education.* New York: Basic Books, 1985.

Ludmerer, Kenneth M. *Time to Heal: American Medical Education from the Turn of the Century to the Era of Managed Care.* New York: Oxford University Press, 1999.

Madrigal, Josef, Sarah Rudasil, Zachary Tran, Jonathan Bergman, and Peyman Benharash. "Sexual and Gender Minority Identity in Undergraduate Medical Education: Impact on Experience and Career Trajectory." *PLOS One* 16, no. 11 (2021): e0260387.

Madzia, Jules L. "Inequality in Medical Professionalization and Specialization." PhD diss., University of Cincinnati, 2023.

Mamdani, Mahmood. "Good Muslim, Bad Muslim: A Political Perspective on Culture and Terrorism." *American Anthropologist* 104, no. 3 (2002): 766–775.

Mann, Sarah. "Focusing on Arts, Humanities to Develop Well-Rounded Physicians." *AAMC News*, August 15. 2017.

Manzer, Jamie L., and Ann V. Bell. "'We're a Little Biased': Medicine and the Management of Bias Through the Case of Contraception. *Journal of Health and Social Behavior* 62, no. 2 (2021): 120–135

Margolis, Eric, and Mary Romero. "The Department Is Very Male, Very White, Very Old, and Very Conservative: The Functioning of the Hidden Curriculum in Graduate Sociology Departments." *Harvard Educational Review* 68, no. 1 (1998): 1–32.

Martimianakis, Maria Athina, Barret Michalec, Justin Lam, Carrie Cartmill, Janelle S. Taylor, and Frederic W. Hafferty. "Humanism, the Hidden Curriculum, and Educational Reform: A Scoping Review and Thematic Analysis." *Academic Medicine* 90, no. 11 (2015): S5–S13.

MacNaughton, Jane. "Medical Humanities' Challenge to Medicine." *Journal of Evaluation in Clinical Practice* 17 (2011): 927–932.

Martinussen, Pål Erling, and Jon Magnussen. "Resisting Market-Inspired Reform in Healthcare: The Role of Professional Subcultures in Medicine." *Social Science and Medicine* 73, no. 2 (2011): 193–200.

McGaghie, William C. "Assessing Readiness for Medical Education: Evolution of the Medical College Admission Test." *Journal of the American Medical Association* 288, no. 9 (2002): 1085–1090.

McKee, Guian. *Hospital City, Healthcare Nation: Race, Capital, and the Costs of American Healthcare*. Philadelphia: University of Pennsylvania Press, 2023.

McKinlay, John B., and Lisa Marceau. "The End of the Golden Age of Doctoring." In *The Sociology of Health and Illness: Critical Perspectives*, 7th ed., ed. Rose Weitz, 189–214. New York: Worth Publishers, 2002.

Mechanic, David. "The Role of Sociology in Health Affairs." *Health Affairs* 9, no. 1 (1990): 85–97.

Medvetz, Thomas. *Think Tanks in America*. Chicago: University of Chicago Press, 2012.

Menand, Louis. *The Marketplace of Ideas: Reform and Resistance in the American University*. New York: W.W. Norton, 2010.

Menchik, Daniel. "Interdependent Career Types and Divergent Standpoints on the Use of Advanced Technology in Medicine." *Journal of Health and Social Behavior* 58, no. 4 (2017): 488–502.

Menchik, Daniel, and David Meltzer. "The Cultivation of Esteem and Retrieval of Scientific Knowledge in Physician Networks." *Journal of Health and Social Behavior* 51, no. 1 (2010): 137–152.

Merton, Robert K., George G. Reader, and Patricia L. Kendall. *The Student-Physician: Introductory Studies in the Sociology of Medical Education*. Cambridge, MA: Harvard University Press, 1957.

Metzl, Jonathan M., and Helena Hansen. "Structural Competency: Theorizing a New Medical Engagement with Stigma and Inequality." *Social Science and Medicine* 103, no. 1 (2014): 126–133.

Meyer, John W., and Brian Rowan. "Institutionalized Organizations: Formal Structure as Myth and Ceremony." *American Journal of Sociology* 83, no. 4 (1977): 340–363.

Michael, Mike, Steven Wainwright, and Clare Williams. "Temporality and Prudence: On Stem Cells as 'Phronesic Things.'" *Configurations* 13, no. 3 (2005): 373–394.

Michalec, Barret, Monica Cuddy, Phillip Hafferty, Mark D. Hanson, Steven L. Kanter, Dawn Littleton, Tina Martimianakis, Robin Michaels, and Frederic W. Hafferty. "It's Happening Sooner Than You Think: Spotlighting the Premedical Realm(s)." *Medical Education* 52, no. 4 (2018): 359–361.

Michalec, Barret, Tina Martimianakis, Jon Tilburt, and Frederic W. Hafferty. "Why It's Unjust to Expect Location-Specific, Language-Specific, or Population-Specific Service from Students with Underrepresented Minority or Low-Income Backgrounds." *AMA Journal of Ethics* 19, no. 3 (2017): 238–244.

Mills, Charles W. *The Racial Contract*. Ithaca, NY: Cornell University Press, 1997.

Moniz, Tracy, Maryam Golafshani, Carolyn M. Gaspar, Nancy E. Adams, Paul Haidet, Javeed Sukhera, Rebecca L. Volpe, Claire de Boer, and Lorelei Lingard. "The Prism Model: Advancing a Theory of Practice for Arts and Humanities in Medical Education." *Perspectives on Medical Education* 10, no. 4 (2021): 207–214.

Moore, Wendy Leo. *Reproducing Racism: White Space, Elite Law Schools, and Racial Inequality*. New York: Rowman and Littlefield, 2008.

Morning, Ann. *The Nature of Race: How Scientists Think and Teach About Human Difference*. Berkeley: University of California Press, 2011.

Morrison, Emory, and Douglas Grbic. "Dimensions of Diversity and Perception of Having Learned from Individuals from Different Backgrounds: The Particular Importance of Racial Diversity." *Academic Medicine* 90, no. 7 (2015): 937–940.

Mueller, Jennifer C. "Racial Ideology or Racial Ignorance? An Alternative Theory of Racial Cognition." *Sociological Theory* 38, no. 2 (2020): 142–169.

Mullan, Fitzhugh. *White Coat, Clenched Fist: The Political Education of an American Physician*. Ann Arbor: University of Michigan Press, 2006.

Murphy, Marie. "Hiding in Plain Sight: The Production of Heteronormativity in Medical Education." *Journal of Contemporary Ethnography* 45, no. 3 (2014): 256–289.

Murphy, Michelle. "Immodest Witnessing: The Epistemology of Vaginal Self-Examination in the U.S. Feminist Self-Help Movement." *Feminist Studies* 30, no. 1 (2004): 115–147.

National Institute of Child Health and Human Development. "Behavioral Sciences and Medical Education: A Report of Four Conferences." DHEW Publication No. (NIH) 72–41, U.S. Department of Health, Education, and Welfare, Public Health Service, National Institutes of Health, 1970.

Nelson, Alondra. *Body and Soul: The Black Panther Party and the Fight Against Medical Discrimination*. Minneapolis: University of Minnesota Press, 2011.

Nguemeni Tiako, Max Jordan, Eugenia C. South, and Victor Ray. "Medical Schools as Racialized Organizations: A Primer." *Annals of Internal Medicine* 174, no. 8 (2022): 1143–1144.

Nguyen, Mytien, Mayur M. Desai, and Tonya L. Fancher. "Temporal Trends in Childhood Household Income Among Applicants and Matriculants to

Medical School and the Likelihood of Acceptance by Income, 2014–2019." *Journal of the American Medical Association* (2023), doi:10.1001/jama.2023.5654.

Nobles, Autumn, Bianka Aceves Martin, Jaileessa Casimir, Sarah Schmitt, and Geoffrey Broadbent. "Stalled Progress: Medical School Dean Demographics." *Journal of the American Board of Family Medicine* 35, no. 1 (2022): 163–168.

Obedin-Maliver, Juno, Elizabeth S. Goldsmith, Leslie Stewart, William White, Eric Tran, Stephanie Brenman, Maggie Wells, David M. Fetterman, Gabriel Garcia, and Mitchell R. Lunn. "Lesbian, Gay, Bisexual, and Transgender–Related Content in Undergraduate Medical Education. *Journal of the American Medical Association* 306, no. 9 (2011): 971–977.

O'Connell, Thomas F., Sandra A. Ham, Theodore G. Hart, Farr A. Curlin, and John D. Yoon. "A National Longitudinal Survey of Medical Students' Intentions to Practice Among the Underserved." *Academic Medicine* 93, no. 1 (2018): 90–97.

O'Connor, Alice. *Poverty Knowledge: Social Science, Social Policy, and the Poor in Twentieth-Century U.S. History*. Princeton, NJ: Princeton University Press, 2001.

Olsen, Lauren D. "'We'd Rather Be Relevant Than Theoretically Accurate': Translational Medicine and the Transmutation of Cultural Anthropology for Clinical Practice." *Social Problems* 68, no. 3 (2021): 761–777.

Olsen, Lauren D., and Hana Gebremariam. "Disciplining Empathy: Differences in Empathy with U.S. Medical Students by College Major." *Health: An Interdisciplinary Journal for the Social Study of Health, Illness and Medicine* 26, no. 4 (2022): 475–494.

Omi, Michael, and Howard Winant. *Racial Formation in the United States: From the 1960s to the 1990s*. New York: Routledge, 1994.

Ong, Maria, Carol Wright, Lorelle L. Espinosa, and Gary Orfield. "Inside the Double Bind: A Synthesis of Empirical Research on Undergraduate and Graduate Women of Color in Science, Technology, Engineering, and Mathematics." *Harvard Educational Review* 81, no. 2 (2011): 172–209.

O'Rourke, Meghan. *The Invisible Kingdom: Reimagining Chronic Illness*. New York: Penguin Books, 2022.

Osman, Magda, Bella Eacott, and Suzy Willson. "Arts-Based Interventions in Healthcare Education." *Medical Humanities* 44, no. 1 (2018): 28–33.

Owens, Deidre Cooper. *Medical Bondage: Race, Gender, and the Origins of American Gynecology*. Athens: University of Georgia Press, 2017.

Padilla, Amado M. "Ethnic Minority Scholars, Research, and Mentoring: Current and Future Issues." *Educational Researcher* 23, no. 4 (1994): 24–27.

Page, Robert Collier. "The Doctor for Tomorrow's Needs." *Journal of the Association of American Medical Colleges* 27, no. 2 (1952): 91–99.

Parker, Palmer. *To Know as We Are Known: Education as a Spiritual Journey.* New York: HarperOne, 1983.

Pedersen, Reidar. "Empathy Development in Medical Education: A Critical Review." *Medical Teaching* 32, no. 7 (2010): 593–600.

Pellegrino, Edmund. "Medical History and Medical Education: Points of Engagement." *Clio Medica* 10, no. 3 (1975): 295–303.

Pellegrino, Edmund. "The Virtuous Physician and the Ethics of Medicine." In *Virtue and Medicine: Explorations in the Character of Medicine,* ed. Earl E. Shelp, 237–255. Dordrecht: Reidel, 1985.

Penfield, Wilder. "Medical School Admissions." *Journal of the Association of American Medical Colleges* 33, no. 7 (1958): 853–855.

Petersdorf, Richard G., and Alvan R. Feinstein. "An Informal Appraisal of the Current Status of 'Medical Sociology.'" *The Relevance of Social Science in Medicine,* ed. Leon Eisenberg and Arthur Kleinman, 27–45. Dordrecht: Reidel, 1981.

Phelan, Sean M., Sara E. Burke, Brooke A. Cunningham, Sylvia P. Perry, Rachel R. Hardeman, John F. Dovidio, Jeph Herrin, Liselotte N. Dyrbye, Richard O. White, Mark W. Yeazel, and Ivuoma N. Onyeador, Natalie M. Wittlin, Kristin Harden, and Michelle van Ryn. "The Effects of Racism in Medical Education on Students' Decisions to Practice in Underserved or Minority Communities." *Academic Medicine* 94, no. 8 (2019): 1178–1189.

Pugh, Allison J. "Emotions and the Systematization of Connective Labor." *Theory, Culture & Society* 39, no. 5 (2021): 23–42.

Quindlen, Anna. *Write for Your Life.* New York: Random House, 2022.

Rabinow, Paul, and Gaymon Bennett. *Designing Human Practices: An Experiment with Synthetic Biology.* Chicago: University of Chicago Press, 2012.

Rabow, Michael W., Marissa Lapedis, Anat Feingold, Mark Thomas, and Rachel N. Remen. "Insisting on the Healer's Art: The Implications of Required Participation in a Medical School Course on Values and Humanism." *Teaching and Learning in Medicine* 28, no. 1 (2016): 61–71.

Ray, Victor. "A Theory of Racialized Organizations." *American Sociological Review* 84, no. 1 (2019): 26–53.

Raz, Aviad, and Judith Fadlon. "'We Came to Talk with the People Behind the Disease': Communication and Control in Medical Education," *Culture, Medicine and Psychiatry* 30, no. 1 (2006): 55–75.

Riess, Helen, and Liz Neporent. *The Empathy Effect: Seven Neuroscience-Based Keys for Transforming the Way We Live, Love, Work, and Connect Across Differences.* Boston: Sounds True Publishing, 2018.

Ripp, Kelsey, and Lundy Braun. "Race/Ethnicity in Medical Education: An Analysis of a Question Bank for Step 1 of the USMLE." *Teaching and Learning in Medicine* 29, no. 2 (2017): 115–122.

Rivera, Lauren A. *Pedigree: How Elite Students Get Elite Jobs.* Princeton, NJ: Princeton University Press, 2015.

Romano, John. "Community Needs: The Student, the Medical School as It Exists Today." *Journal of Medical Education* 27, no. 3 (1952): 168–169.

Rylance, Rick. *Literature and the Public Good.* New York: Oxford University Press, 2010.

Saunders, Barry F., and Lundy Braun. "Reforming the Use of Race in Medical Pedagogy." *American Journal of Bioethics* 17, no. 9 (2017): 50–52.

Seamster, Louise, and Victor Ray. "Against Teleology in the Study of Race: Toward the Abolition of the Progress Paradigm." *Sociological Theory* 36, no. 4 (2018): 315–342.

Seim, Josh. *Bandage, Sort, and Hustle: Ambulance Crews on the Front Lines of Urban Suffering.* Berkeley: University of California Press, 2020.

Shanafelt, Tait D., Omar Hasan, Liselotte N. Dyrbye, Christine Sinksy, Daniel Satele, Jeff Sloan, and Colin P. West. "Changes in Burnout and Satisfaction with Work-Life Balance in Physicians and the General U.S. Working Population Between 2011 and 2014." *Mayo Clinic Proceedings* 90, no. 12 (2015): 1600–1613.

Sharfstein, Steven S. "Big Pharma and American Psychiatry: The Good, the Bad, and the Ugly." *Psychiatric News* August 19, 2005. doi:10.1176/pn.40.16.00400003.

Sharma, Malika, and Ayelet Kuper. "The Elephant in the Room: Talking Race in Medical Education." *Advances in Health Sciences Education* 22, no. 3 (2017): 761–764.

Sharma, Malika, Andrew D. Pinto, Arno K. Kumagai. "Teaching the Social Determinants of Health: A Path to Equity or a Road to Nowhere?" *Academic Medicine* 93, no. 1 (2018): 25–30.

Shim, Janet K. *Heart-Sick: The Politics of Risk, Inequality, and Heart Disease.* New York: New York University Press, 2014.

shuster, stef m. *Trans Medicine: The Emergence and Practice of Treating Gender.* New York: New York University Press, 2021.

Sidney, Sir Philip. "The Defense of Poesy." In *The Defense of Poesy Otherwise Known as an Apology for Poetry,* ed. Albert S. Cook. Boston: Ginn, 1890.

Sierra-Arevalo, Michael. *The Danger Imperative: Violence, Death, and the Soul of Policing.* New York: Columbia University Press, 2024.

Sigerist, Henry. "Medical History in the Medical Schools of the United States." *Bulletin of the History of Medicine* 7, no. 6 (1939): 627–662.

Silverman, Arielle. *Just Human: The Quest for Disability, Wisdom, Respect, and Inclusion*. Baltimore: Disability Wisdom Publishing, 2021.

Skorton, David, and Ashley Bear. *The Integration of the Humanities and Arts with Sciences, Engineering, and Medicine in Higher Education: Branches from the Same Tree*. Washington, DC: National Academy of Sciences, 2018.

Small, Helen H. *The Value of the Humanities*. New York: Oxford University Press, 2016.

Smedley, Brian D., Adrienne Y. Stith, Alan R. Nelson, and Institute of Medicine (U.S.) Committee on Understanding and Eliminating Racial and Ethnic Disparities in Health Care. *Unequal Treatment: Confronting Racial and Ethnic Disparities in Health Care*. Washington, DC: National Academy Press, 2003.

Smyth, Francis Scott. "The Place of the Humanities and Social Sciences in the Education of Physicians." *Journal of Medical Education* 37, no. 5 (1962): 495–499.

Sointu, Eeva. "'Good' Patient/'Bad' Patient: Clinical Learning and the Entrenching of Inequality." *Sociology of Health and Illness* 39, no. 1 (2017): 63–77.

Starr, Paul. *The Social Transformation of American Medicine*. New York: Basic Books, 1982.

Steinmetz, George. *The Politics of Method in the Human Sciences: Positivism and Its Epistemological Others*. Durham, NC: Duke University Press, 2005.

Stepanikova, Irena. "Racial-Ethnic Biases, Time Pressure, and Medical Decisions." *Journal of Health and Social Behavior* 53, no. 3 (2010): 329–343.

Stevens, Mitchell L. *Creating a Class: College Admissions and the Education of Elites*. Cambridge, MA: Harvard University Press, 2007.

Stevens, Mitchell L., Elizabeth Armstrong, and Richard Arum. "Sieve, Incubator, Temple, Hub: Empirical and Conceptual Advances in the Sociology of Higher Education." *Annual Review of Sociology* 34 (2008): 127–151.

Stiles, William W., Francis Scott Smyth, and Mathea Reuter, "Individual and Community Health Instruction in the Premedical Curriculum," *Journal of Medical Education* 28, no. 6 (1953): 29.

Stonington, Scott D., Seth M. Holmes, Helena Hansen, Jeremy A. Green, Keith A. Wailoo, Debra Malina, Stephen Morrissey, Paul E. Farmer, and Michael G. Marmot. "Case Studies in Social Medicine: Attending to Structural Forces in Clinical Practice." *New England Journal of Medicine* 379, no. 19 (2018): 1958–1961.

Taylor, Janelle. "Confronting 'Culture' in Medicine's 'Culture of No Culture.'" *Academic Medicine* 7, no. 6 (2003): 555–559.

Torres, Lucas, Mark W. Driscoll, and Anthony L. Burrow. "Racial Microaggressions and Psychological Functioning Among Highly Achieving African-Americans:

A Mixed-Methods Approach." *Journal of Social and Clinical Psychology* 29, no. 10 (2010): 1074–1099.

Touya de Marienne, Eric. *The Case for the Humanities: Pedagogy, Polity, and Interdisciplinarity.* Baltimore, MD: Rowman and Littlefield, 2016.

Trotter, LaTonya J. "A Dream Deferred: Professional Projects as Racial Projects in US Medicine." In *The Routledge Handbook on the American Dream,* ed. Robert C. Hauhart and Mitja Sardoc, 331–351. New York: Routledge, 2022.

Trotter, LaTonya J. Keynote address at a preconference on the Social Transformation of the Sociology of Health Professions Education at the American Sociological Association annual meeting. August 17, 2023.

Trow, Martin. "The Campus as a Context for Learning." In *Martin Trow: Twentieth-Century Higher Education: Elite to Mass to Universal,* ed. Michael Burrage, 303–318. Baltimore, MD: Johns Hopkins University Press, 2010.

Tsai, Jennifer, Neil Baldwin, Laura Ucik, Christopher Hasslinger, and George Paul. "Race Matters? Examining and Rethinking Race Portrayal in Preclinical Medical Education." *Academic Medicine* 91, no. 7 (2016): 916–920.

Jennifer Tsai, Edwin Lindo, and Khiara Bridges. "Seeing the Window, Finding the Spider: Applying Critical Race Theory to Medical Education to Make Up Where Biomedical Models and Social Determinants of Health Curricula Fall Short." *Frontiers in Public Health* 9 (2021): 1–10.

Tweedy, Damon. *Black Man in a White Coat.* New York: Picador, 2015.

Tyler, David B. "A University is an Institution That Has Trouble with Its Medical School." *Journal of Medical Education* 35, no. 8 (1960): 791–795.

Tzreciak, Stephen, and Anthony Mazzarelli. *Compassionomics: The Revolutionary Scientific Evidence That Caring Makes a Difference.* New York: Studer Group, 2019.

Underman, Kelly. "Burnout Inventories and the Unsettled Science of Wellness in Health Professions Education." BeSST Conference. Edinburgh, August 17, 2023.

Underman, Kelly. *Feeling Medicine: How the Pelvic Exam Shapes Medical Training.* New York: New York University Press, 2020.

Underman, Kelly. "Playing Doctor: Simulation in Medical School as Affective Practice." *Social Science and Medicine* 136, no. 1 (2015): 180–188.

Underman, Kelly, and Laura E. Hirshfield. "Detached Concern? Emotional Socialization in Twenty-First Century Medical Education." *Social Science and Medicine* 160, no. 1 (2016): 94–101.

van Ryn, Michelle, Diana J. Burgess, John F. Dovidio, Sean M. Phelan, Somnath Saha, Jennifer Malat, Joan M. Griffin, Steven S. Fu, and Sylvia Perry. "The Impact of Racism on Clinician Cognition, Behavior, and Clinical Decision Making." *DuBois Review* 8, no. 1 (2011): 199–218.

van Ryn, Michelle, and Steven S. Fu. "Paved with Good Intentions: Do Public Health and Human Service Providers Contribute to Racial/Ethnic Disparities in Health?" *American Journal of Public Health* 93, no. 2 (2003): 248–255.

van Ryn, Michelle, Rachel Hardeman, Sean M. Phelan, Diana J. Burgess, John F. Dovidio, Jeph Herrin, Sara E. Burke, David B. Nelson, Sylvi Perry, Mark Yeazel, and Julia M. Przedworski. "Medical School Experiences Associated with Change in Implicit Racial Bias Among 3547 Students: A Medical Student CHANGES Study Report." *Journal of General Internal Medicine* 30, no. 12 (2015): 1748–1756.

Vaughan, Diane. *The Challenger Launch Decision: Risky Technology, Culture, and Deviance at NASA.* Chicago: University of Chicago Press, 1996.

Velasquez, David E., Arman A. Shahriar, and Fidencio Saldana. "Economic Disparity and the Physician Pipeline—Medicine's Uphill Battle." *Journal of General Internal Medicine* 2023. doi:10.1007/s11606-023-08109-3.

Villarosa, Linda. *Under the Skin: The Hidden Toll of Racism on American Lives and on the Health of Our Nation.* New York: Anchor, 2023.

Vinson, Alexandra H. "'Constrained Collaboration': Patient Empowerment Discourse as Resource for Countervailing Power." *Sociology of Health and Illness* 38, no. 8 (2016): 1364–1378.

Vinson, Alexandra H. "Short White Coats: Knowledge, Identity, and Status Negotiations of First-Year Medical Students." *Symbolic Interaction* 42, no. 3 (2019): 395–411.

Vinson, Alexandra H. "Teaching the Work of Doctoring: How the Medical Profession Adapts to Change." PhD diss., University of California San Diego, 2015.

Vinson, Alexandra H., and Kelly Underman. "Clinical Empathy as Emotional Labor in Medical Work." *Social Science and Medicine* 251 (2020): 1–9.

Viseu, Ana. "Caring for Nanotechnology? Being an Integrated Social Scientist." *Social Studies of Science* 45, no. 5 (2015): 625–664.

Waitzkin, Howard. "Changing Patient-Physician Relationships in the Changing Health-Policy Environment." In *Handbook of Medical Sociology*, ed. Chloe Bird, Peter Conrad, and Allen Fremont, 271–283. Upper Saddle River. NJ: Prentice-Hall, 2000.

Waitzkin, Howard. *Politics of Medical Encounters: How Patients and Doctors Deal with Social Problems.* New Haven, CT: Yale University Press, 1991.

Warikoo, Natasha K. *The Diversity Bargain: And Other Dilemmas of Race, Admissions, and Meritocracy at Elite Universities.* Chicago: University of Chicago Press, 2016.

Waring, Justin, Fiona Marshall, Simon Bishop, Opinder Sahota, Marion Walker, Graeme Currie, Rebecca Fisher, and Tony Avery. *An Ethnographic Study of*

Knowledge Sharing Across the Boundaries Between Care Processes, Services, and Organizations: The Contributions to 'Safe' Hospital Discharge. Health Services and Delivery Research No. 2.29. London: National Institute for Health Research, 2014.

Warraich, Haider. *The Song of Our Scars: The Untold Story of Pain.* New York: Basic Books, 2022.

Wear, Delese. "Insurgent Multiculturalism: Rethinking How and Why We Teach Culture in Medical Education." *Academic Medicine* 78, no. 6 (2003): 549–554.

Wear, Delese, Joseph Zarconi, Arno Kumagai, and Kathy Cole-Kelly. "Slow Medical Education." *Academic Medicine* 90, no. 3 (2015): 289–293.

Weaver, Warren. "Medicine: The New Science and the Old Art." *Journal of Medical Education* 35, no. 4 (1960): 313–318.

Wegar, Katarina. "Sociology in American Medical Education Since the 1960s: The Rhetoric of Reform." *Social Science and Medicine* 35, no. 8 (1992): 959–965.

West, Colin P., Tait D. Shanafelt, and Joseph C. Kolars. "Quality of Life, Burnout, Educational Debt, and Medical Knowledge Among Internal Medicine Residents." *Journal of the American Medical Association* 306, no. 9 (2011): 952–960.

White Coats 4 Black Lives. "Racial Justice Report Card." Accessed May 4, 2018. http://whitecoats4blacklives.org/wp-content/uploads/2018/04/WC4BL -Racial-Justice-Report-Card-2018-Full-Report-2.pdf.

Whitehead, Anne, and Angela Woods. *The Edinburgh Companion to the Critical Medical Humanities.* Edinburgh: Edinburgh University Press, 2016.

Whitehead, Cynthia R., Brian D. Hodges, and Zubin Austin. "Captive on a Carousel: Discourses of 'New' in Medical Education 1910–2010." *Advances in Health Sciences Education* 18 (2013): 755–768.

Whitehead, Cynthia R., Brian D. Hodges, and Zubin Austin. "Dissecting the Doctor: From Character to Characteristics in North American Medical Education." *Advances in Health Sciences Education* 18 (2013): 687–699.

Willard, William R. "New Medical Schools: Some Preliminary Considerations." *Journal of Medical Education* 35, no. 2 (1960): 95–107.

Williams, David R. "Miles to Go Before We Sleep: Racial Inequalities in Health." *Journal of Health and Social Behavior* 53, no. 3 (2012): 279–295.

Williams, Stacy J., Laura Pecenco, and Mary Blair-Loy. *Medical Professions: The Status of Women and Men.* La Jolla, CA: University of California San Diego, 2013.

Willoughby, Christopher. *Masters of Health: Racial Sciences and Slavery in U.S. Medical Schools.* Raleigh: University of North Carolina Press, 2022.

Wingfield, Adia Harvey. *Flatlining: Race, Work, and Health Care in the New Economy.* Berkeley: University of California Press, 2019.

Wong, Sarah H. M., Faye Gishen, and Amali U. Lokugamage. "'Decolonizing the Medical Curriculum': Humanizing Medicine Through Epistemic Pluralism, Cultural Safety, and Critical Consciousness." *London Review of Education* 19, no. 1 (2021). doi:10.14324/LRE.19.1.16.

Yu, Peter T., Pouria V. Parsa, Omar Hassanein, Selwyn O. Rogers, and David C. Chang. "Minorities Struggle to Advance in Academic Medicine: A 12-Year Review of Diversity at the Highest Levels of America's Teaching Institutions." *Journal of Surgical Residency* 182, no. 2 (2013): 212–218.

Zusman, Ami. "Challenges Facing Higher Education in the Twenty-First Century." In *American Higher Education in the Twenty-First Century*, ed. Philip G. Altbach, Robert O. Berdahl, and Patricia J. Gumport, 115–160. Baltimore, MD: Johns Hopkins University Press, 2005.

INDEX

Page numbers in *italics* refer to tables.

Printed and bound by CPI Group (UK) Ltd, Croydon, CR0 4YY

28/10/2024

14581409-0001